Diverticulitis Cookbook

Embrace Nutritious, Easy-to-Make Recipes to Heal Your Gut, Enhance Wellness, and Bring Delight to Every Mealtime

Avery Lynn Morgan

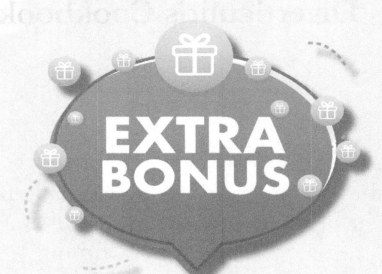
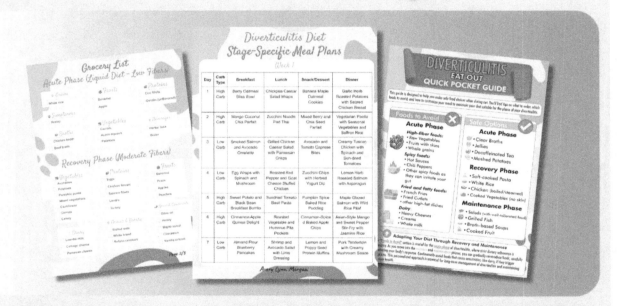

INSIDE THE BOOK

STAGE-SPECIFIC MEAL PLANS
PHASE-TAILORED GROCERY LIST
EAT OUT QUICK POCKET GUIDE
All printable in FULL COLOR

Scroll to the end and **SCAN** the **QR CODE**

© Copyright 2024 Avery Lynn Morgan all rights reserved.

This document is geared towards providing exact and reliable information with regard to the topic and issue covered. The publication is sold with the idea that the publisher is not required to render accounting, officially permitted, or otherwise qualified services. If advice is necessary, legal or professional, a practiced individual in the profession should be ordered.

From a Declaration of Principles which was accepted and approved equally by a Committee of the American Bar Association and a Committee of Publishers and Associations.

In no way is it legal to reproduce, duplicate, or transmit any part of this document in either electronic means or in printed format. Recording of this publication is strictly prohibited, and any storage of this document is not allowed unless with written permission from the publisher. All rights reserved.

The information provided herein is stated to be truthful and consistent, in that any liability, in terms of inattention or otherwise, by any usage or abuse of any policies, processes, or directions contained within is the solitary and utter responsibility of the recipient reader. Under no circumstances will any legal responsibility or blame be held against the publisher for any reparation, damages, or monetary loss due to the information herein, either directly or indirectly.

Table of Contents

INTRODUCTION 8

PART I: UNDERSTANDING DIVERTICULITIS AND ITS DIETARY MANAGEMENT 9

CHAPTER 1:   DIVERTICULITIS DEMYSTIFIED.. 9

UNDERSTANDING DIVERTICULITIS.. 9
SYMPTOMS AND CAUSES 10
THE ROLE OF DIET IN MANAGEMENT 10
NAVIGATING YOUR DIET THROUGH THE STAGES OF DIVERTICULITIS 10

CHAPTER 2:   NAVIGATING YOUR DIET THROUGH THE STAGES OF DIVERTICULITIS 12

A JOURNEY OF ADAPTATION.. 12
THE ACUTE PHASE: CRISIS MANAGEMENT... 12
THE RECOVERY PHASE: BUILDING STRENGTH 12
THE MAINTENANCE PHASE: PREVENTION AND PROSPERITY 13
TAILORING YOUR DIET TO YOUR JOURNEY 13

PART II: RECIPES FOR EACH STAGE OF DIVERTICULITIS 14

CHAPTER 3:   ACUTE PHASE: CLEAR LIQUID AND LOW-FIBER RECIPES 14

BREAKFAST RECIPES 15
    1.   *Gentle Ginger Tea* 15
    2.   *Clear Chicken Broth* 15
    3.   *Soothing Rice Porridge*... 16
    4.   *Basic Apple Gelatin* 16
    5.   *Herbal Infusion Blend* 17
    6.   *Plain Rice Water* 17
    7.   *Low-Fiber Cream of Wheat*.. 18
    8.   *Simple Poached Pear* 18
    9.   *Bland Scrambled Egg Whites* 19
    10.   *Steamed White Rice Mash* 19

SNACK RECIPES 20
    11.   *Soothing Clear Broth Cubes* 20
    12.   *Gentle Apple and Cinnamon Compote* 20
    13.   *Hydrating Herbal Ice Pops* 21
    14.   *Cooling Peppermint Tea Gelatin* 21
    15.   *Simple Honey-Drizzled Poached Pears* 22

LUNCH RECIPES 23
    16.   *Broth-Based Vegetable Soup* 23
    17.   *Mashed Carrot Puree* 23
    18.   *Tender Chicken Broth Soup*... 24
    19.   *Soft-Cooked Acorn Squash*... 25
    20.   *Plain Gelatin Cups* 25
    21.   *Silky Potato Soup* 26
    22.   *Low-Fiber Baked Apple* 26
    23.   *Clear Beef Broth* 27
    24.   *Simple Poached Chicken Breast* 28
    25.   *Pureed Pumpkin Soup* 28

DINNER RECIPES 30
    26.   *Butternut Squash Puree*.. 30
    27.   *Strained Lentil Soup*... 30
    28.   *Steamed White Fish Fillet* 31
    29.   *Baked Sweet Potato Mash* 32
    30.   *Clear Tomato Broth* 32
    31.   *Low-Fiber Turkey Soup* 33

32.	Gentle Zucchini Soup	34
33.	Plain Gelatin with Fruit Juice	35
34.	Poached Cod in Broth	35
35.	Smooth Carrot and Ginger Soup	36

CHAPTER 4:   RECOVERY PHASE: LOW TO MODERATE FIBER RECIPES 37

BREAKFAST RECIPES 38

36.	Creamy Oatmeal with Mashed Banana	38
37.	Scrambled Eggs with Avocado	38
38.	Baked Pears with Honey	39
39.	Cottage Cheese with Soft Peaches	40
40.	Smooth Peanut Butter on Toasted White Bread	40
41.	Rice Porridge with Maple Syrup	41
42.	Mashed Pumpkin Pancakes	41
43.	Soft-Boiled Eggs with Saltine Crackers	42
44.	Low-Fiber Blueberry Muffins	42
45.	Applesauce with Cinnamon Yogurt	43

SNACK RECIPES 44

46.	Mild Avocado Mash on Toasted White Bread	44
47.	Baked Banana with a Dash of Cinnamon	44
48.	Creamy Low-Fiber Pumpkin Smoothie	45
49.	Soft-Cooked Apple and Pear Sauce	45
50.	Low-Fiber Berry and Yogurt Parfait	46

LUNCH RECIPES 47

51.	Quinoa Salad with Roasted Vegetables	47
52.	Baked Sweet Potato with Cottage Cheese	48
53.	Pureed Butternut Squash Soup	48
54.	Soft-Cooked Chicken and Rice Bowl	49
55.	Steamed Salmon with Mashed Cauliflower	50
56.	Turkey and Avocado Wrap with Soft Tortilla	50
57.	Low-Fiber Vegetable Stir-Fry with Tofu	51
58.	Pumpkin Soup with a Dollop of Greek Yogurt	52
59.	Soft-Cooked Pasta with Olive Oil and Parmesan	53
60.	Lentil Stew with Carrots and Celery	53

DINNER RECIPES 55

61.	Grilled Tilapia with Lemon Herb Dressing	55
62.	Roasted Carrot and Ginger Soup	56
63.	Baked Cod with Soft Herbed Polenta	57
64.	Turkey Meatballs in Low-Fiber Tomato Sauce	57
65.	Soft-Cooked Vegetable Quiche without Crust	58
66.	Poached Pear Salad with Walnut Dressing	59
67.	Mashed Root Vegetables with Grilled Chicken Breast	60
68.	Creamy Risotto with Parmesan and Spinach	61
69.	Stewed Beef with Pumpkin Puree	62
70.	Broccoli and Cauliflower Cheese Bake	63

CHAPTER 5:   MAINTENANCE PHASE: HIGH-FIBER RECIPES 64

BREAKFAST RECIPES 65

71.	Mixed Berry and Chia Seed Parfait	65
72.	Whole Grain Toast with Avocado Spread	65
73.	Oatmeal with Fresh Fruit and Almonds	66
74.	Spinach and Feta Whole Wheat Muffins	67
75.	Quinoa Breakfast Bowl with Berries	68
76.	Whole Grain Pancakes with Maple Syrup	68
77.	Baked Sweet Potato and Black Bean Hash	69

78.	Greek Yogurt Smoothie with Mixed Berries	70
79.	Vegetable and Goat Cheese Frittata	71
80.	Banana and Walnut Whole Wheat Bread	72

SNACK RECIPES 73
81.	Crunchy Chickpea and Kale Chips	73
82.	Almond and Flaxseed Energy Balls	73
83.	Whole Grain Crackers with Spicy Hummus	74
84.	Fresh Veggie Sticks with Avocado Dip	74
85.	Raspberry and Chia Seed Pudding	75

LUNCH RECIPES 76
86.	Mediterranean Quinoa Salad with Chickpeas	76
87.	Grilled Chicken Caesar Wrap with Whole Wheat Tortilla	77
88.	Roasted Vegetable and Hummus Pita Pockets	78
89.	Kale and Quinoa Salad with Lemon Tahini Dressing	78
90.	Turkey and Avocado Club Sandwich on Multigrain Bread	79
91.	Black Bean and Corn Taco Salad with Whole Grain Chips	80
92.	Whole Wheat Pasta Salad with Cherry Tomatoes and Feta	81
93.	Asian-inspired Tofu and Vegetable Stir Fry	82
94.	Lentil Soup with Spinach and Carrots	83
95.	Grilled Salmon Salad with Mixed Greens and Vinaigrette	84

DINNER RECIPES 85
96.	Stuffed Bell Peppers with Brown Rice and Turkey	85
97.	Eggplant and Chickpea Curry with Quinoa	86
98.	Roasted Butternut Squash and Lentil Salad	87
99.	Baked Trout with Walnut and Herb Crust	88
100.	Vegetarian Black Bean Enchiladas	89
101.	Garlic Ginger Stir-Fried Vegetables with Tempeh	90
102.	Spaghetti Squash with Chunky Tomato Sauce and Olives	91
103.	Moroccan-Spiced Chicken with Couscous and Vegetables	91
104.	Zucchini Noodles with Avocado Pesto and Cherry Tomatoes	93
105.	Portobello Mushroom Steaks with Barley Pilaf	94

PART III: SPECIALIZED DIETARY CONSIDERATIONS AND MEAL PLANNING 95

CHAPTER 6:   CREATING YOUR DIVERTICULITIS DIET PLAN 95

UNDERSTANDING YOUR BODY 95
PERSONALIZING YOUR DIET PLAN 95
INCORPORATING VARIETY AND NUTRITION 95
SUPPLEMENTATION AND DIVERTICULITIS 95
LIFESTYLE CONSIDERATIONS 95
EATING OUT AND SOCIAL EVENTS 96
ADJUSTING AND EVOLVING YOUR DIET PLAN 96
NOURISH & FLOURISH: 7-DAY DIVERTICULITIS DIET PLANS 96

CHAPTER 7:   RECIPES THAT ADAPT WITH YOU 100

ADAPTABLE FOUNDATION RECIPES: THE HEART OF FLEXIBILITY 100
TAILORING TEXTURES AND FLAVORS 100
PHASE-SPECIFIC RECIPE ADAPTATIONS: NAVIGATING THE JOURNEY 100
PERSONALIZING YOUR PLATE: THE ULTIMATE GOAL 100

PART IV: LIVING WELL WITH DIVERTICULITIS 101

CHAPTER 8:   BEYOND DIET: LIFESTYLE CHANGES FOR DIVERTICULITIS MANAGEMENT 101

INTRODUCTION: HOLISTIC HEALTH FOR HOLISTIC HEALING 101
STRESS MANAGEMENT: SOOTHING THE MIND TO SOOTHE THE GUT 101
PHYSICAL ACTIVITY: KEEPING THE BODY MOVING 101

SLEEP AND REST: FOUNDATIONS OF HEALING 101
HYDRATION: THE ESSENCE OF DIGESTIVE HEALTH 101
COMMUNITY AND SUPPORT: NAVIGATING TOGETHER 101
A LIFESTYLE ALIGNED 102

CHAPTER 9:   NAVIGATING CHALLENGES: DINING OUT AND SOCIAL EVENTS 103

INTRODUCTION: EMBRACING SOCIAL LIFE WITH CONFIDENCE 103
PREPARING FOR DINING OUT 103
MANAGING SOCIAL GATHERINGS 103
ALCOHOL AND BEVERAGES 103
NAVIGATING BUFFETS AND POTLUCKS 103
BUILDING RESILIENCE 103
THRIVING SOCIALLY WITH DIVERTICULITIS 104

CONCLUSION 105

EMPOWERING YOUR JOURNEY WITH KNOWLEDGE AND FLAVOR 105

APPENDICES 106

APPENDIX A: FOOD DIARY TEMPLATE: TO TRACK SYMPTOMS AND IDENTIFY TRIGGER FOODS 106
DAILY FOOD DIARY TEMPLATE 106
TIPS FOR KEEPING A FOOD DIARY 106
APPENDIX B: QUICK REFERENCE GUIDE FOR STAGE-SPECIFIC FOODS 107
ACUTE PHASE: SOOTHING AND GENTLE 107
RECOVERY PHASE: GRADUAL REINTRODUCTION 107
MAINTENANCE PHASE: DIVERSE AND BALANCED 107

Introduction

Welcome to "Diverticulitis Cookbook for Beginners: Embrace Nutritious, Easy-to-Make Recipes to Heal Your Gut, Enhance Wellness, and Bring Delight to Every Mealtime." This book is a beacon of hope and a source of empowerment for those navigating the complexities of diverticulitis, offering a path toward a healthier, more enjoyable culinary journey.

Diverticulitis, characterized by its unpredictable flare-ups and periods of remission, challenges individuals not just physically but also emotionally and socially, turning what should be one of life's simple pleasures—eating—into a complex, often stressful endeavor. It transcends the mere objective of symptom management or pain avoidance. This condition invites a deeper introspection into how we nourish our bodies, how we can still find joy and satisfaction in our meals, and importantly, how food can continue to be a source of connection with our loved ones.

This cookbook acknowledges the multifaceted impact of diverticulitis. It aims to serve not only as a guide through the turbulent waters of dietary restrictions but as a beacon of hope for those seeking to reclaim their love for food. It's crafted to arm you with comprehensive knowledge about the nature of diverticulitis and its dietary implications, detailed tools for navigating each stage of the condition, and a collection of recipes designed to meet your nutritional needs without sacrificing flavor or diversity.

Here, the journey through each phase of diverticulitis is demystified, offering a clear path towards maintaining a balanced, gut-friendly diet that supports your health and wellness. From soothing meals that provide comfort during flare-ups to nutrient-rich dishes that promote gut health during remission, each recipe is more than a meal; it's a step towards healing. This approach doesn't just focus on the individual—it encompasses the whole family, ensuring that meals can be enjoyed together, fostering connection and understanding within the family unit.

By integrating practical meal planning and preparation strategies, alongside advice for adapting to the social aspects of dining and managing dietary changes over time, this book aims to simplify living with diverticulitis. It's a testament to the fact that a diverticulitis diagnosis doesn't have to mean the end of enjoyable eating. Instead, it can be the beginning of a new, informed approach to food that prioritizes your health and happiness, allowing you to live well with diverticulitis.

So, this book is more than just about what to eat. It's about embracing a lifestyle that supports your digestive health. We'll explore how to plan and prepare meals efficiently, how to make smart choices when dining out, and how to adjust your diet as your needs change. Through practical advice and personal insights, we aim to make living with diverticulitis more manageable and less intimidating.

Our goal is to empower you to take control of your health through diet. Whether you're newly diagnosed, seeking to prevent flare-ups, or somewhere in between, this cookbook is your companion on the road to wellness. It's not just about managing symptoms—it's about enhancing your overall quality of life, one meal at a time.

Join us as we embark on this journey together, transforming the challenges of diverticulitis into opportunities for healing, enjoyment, and culinary discovery.

Part I: Understanding Diverticulitis and Its Dietary Management

Chapter 1: Diverticulitis Demystified

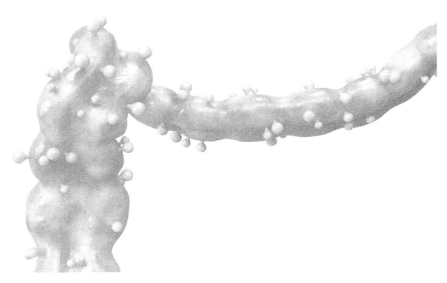

Understanding Diverticulitis

Diverticulitis marks a profound turning point in the way individuals perceive and interact with food and their overall health. This condition, characterized by the inflammation of diverticula—tiny, sac-like protrusions in the lining of the digestive tract—can transform one's diet from a matter of preference to a matter of necessity. Diverticulosis, the presence of these pouches without associated symptoms, is relatively common, particularly as people age. However, when these pouches become inflamed, leading to diverticulitis, the situation changes drastically.

The progression from asymptomatic diverticulosis to symptomatic diverticulitis can occur without warning, ushering in a range of symptoms that can dramatically affect daily life. These symptoms may vary widely in their intensity, from mild discomfort and bloating to severe abdominal pain, fever, and significant changes in bowel habits. Such symptoms not only demand immediate medical attention but also necessitate a reevaluation of one's dietary habits and preferences.

The shift to a diet that accommodates and mitigates the symptoms of diverticulitis often involves significant adjustments. Initially, during acute flare-ups, a highly restrictive diet may be required, typically starting with clear liquids to minimize strain on the digestive system. As symptoms subside, a gradual reintroduction of solid foods begins, with a focus on low-fiber options that are easier to digest. Over time, and particularly during periods of remission, a high-fiber diet is recommended to help prevent future episodes. This long-term dietary strategy aims not just at symptom management but at fostering a healthier, more resilient digestive tract.

These dietary adjustments underscore the need for individuals with diverticulitis to develop a new relationship with food—one that prioritizes nutritional value, digestive comfort, and the preventive management of symptoms over mere taste preferences. This shift is not just about eliminating certain foods or adding others; it's about a holistic approach to eating that considers the timing of meals, the balance of nutrients, and the body's response to different types of food.

Living with diverticulitis, therefore, involves a continuous process of learning and adaptation. It requires individuals to become keen observers of their bodies, to understand the triggers that may precipitate a flare-up, and to navigate the complexities of nutritional science in practical, everyday meal planning. This evolution in the approach to eating and health is not merely a response to a medical condition but an opportunity to cultivate a more mindful, intentional relationship with food, one that enhances quality of life and well-being despite the challenges posed by diverticulitis.

Symptoms and Causes

The pathway to comprehending diverticulitis unfolds as we begin to identify its hallmark symptoms. These symptoms are not merely physical discomforts but signals from the body indicating deeper issues within the digestive tract. Abdominal pain, often sharp and specific to the lower left side, heralds the onset, accompanied by fever that suggests an inflammatory response. Gastrointestinal upset, ranging from nausea to severe changes in bowel habits, including constipation or diarrhea, further complicates the clinical picture, emphasizing the disruption to the digestive system's normal functioning.

Exploring the causes of diverticulitis unveils a complex interplay of factors that go beyond mere chance. Genetic predisposition plays a non-negligible role, suggesting that family history can predispose individuals to this condition, underscoring an inherited vulnerability in the structure or function of the digestive system. Lifestyle choices, particularly those related to diet, exercise, and overall gut health, emerge as pivotal in either mitigating or exacerbating this predisposition. Diets low in fiber have been implicated in contributing to the formation of diverticula by increasing colon pressure, necessitating harder contractions to move small, hard stools.

Moreover, the sedentary lifestyle, common in today's society, may further increase risk, as physical activity is known to promote regular bowel movements and overall digestive health. Additionally, smoking, excessive use of non-steroidal anti-inflammatory drugs (NSAIDs), and obesity are identified as risk factors, weaving a tapestry of lifestyle elements that, when mismanaged, pave the way for diverticulitis to take hold.

This complex etiology of diverticulitis, where genetic, dietary, and lifestyle factors intertwine, illuminates the need for a holistic management strategy. Such an approach transcends the boundaries of conventional medical treatment, advocating for significant lifestyle adjustments alongside medical guidance. It calls for a comprehensive reevaluation of dietary habits, with an emphasis on increasing fiber intake to soften stools and decrease colon pressure. Regular physical activity becomes a cornerstone of prevention, encouraging bowel regularity and contributing to overall weight management. Moreover, understanding and modifying these risk factors can empower individuals to take proactive steps toward not only managing symptoms but also preventing the progression of the disease.

Thus, the journey through understanding and managing diverticulitis is multifaceted, demanding attention to the body's signals, an understanding of the condition's roots, and a commitment to adopting a lifestyle that supports gut health and overall well-being.

The Role of Diet in Management

The intersection of diet and diverticulitis management is a crucial focus. The transition from a standard to a diverticulitis-conscious diet hinges on the condition's phases. Initially, during acute flare-ups, the goal is to minimize bowel activity with a clear liquid diet, gradually transitioning to low-fiber foods as symptoms begin to subside.

Navigating Your Diet Through the Stages of Diverticulitis

Managing your diet through the various stages of diverticulitis requires a nuanced approach, blending mindfulness with strategic dietary planning. This journey through dietary management is not static but dynamic, evolving in response to the body's needs as it moves through different phases of diverticulitis.

- **During Flare-Ups**: In this acute phase, the digestive system demands rest and gentleness. The pivot towards a minimalist diet, comprising broths, teas, and clear juices, is designed to soothe the digestive tract while minimizing any strain. These simple, easily digestible liquids provide the body with hydration and essential nutrients without taxing the digestive system. This dietary approach not only aims to alleviate the immediate discomfort and inflammation but also primes the body for the healing process. By reducing digestive workload, we create an environment conducive to recovery, allowing the inflamed diverticula to heal.
- **Post-Flare-Up Recovery**: As the acute symptoms of a flare-up recede, the dietary focus shifts towards rebuilding and strengthening the digestive system. The gradual reintroduction of fiber marks this phase, beginning with low-fiber foods that are gentle on the gut, such as cooked vegetables, ripe fruits, and soft grains. This cautious approach ensures that while the body begins to readjust to more substantial foods, it is not overwhelmed. The goal is to incrementally increase fiber intake, monitoring the body's response closely and adjusting as needed to prevent any recurrence of symptoms. This phase is pivotal, as it bridges the gap between healing from an acute episode and returning to a diet that supports long-term digestive health.
- **Long-Term Management**: The cornerstone of long-term diverticulitis management is the prevention of future flare-ups, achieved through a diet rich in dietary fiber. However, this involves more than merely

increasing the quantity of fruits and vegetables consumed. It necessitates a holistic understanding of dietary fiber, differentiating between soluble and insoluble fibers, and how they each contribute to digestive health. Adequate hydration is paramount, as water works in tandem with fiber to facilitate smooth bowel movements. Moreover, the timing of meals and the balance of food groups play crucial roles in maintaining digestive harmony. This comprehensive approach to diet underscores the importance of not just what is eaten, but how and when, ensuring that the digestive system is supported without being overloaded.

Each stage in the management of diverticulitis underscores the importance of dietary adaptation and balance. By attentively navigating these dietary phases, individuals can effectively manage their condition, reducing the likelihood of flare-ups and promoting overall digestive health. This journey through diverticulitis is deeply personal, requiring individuals to become attuned to their bodies' signals and responses to different foods, fostering a relationship with food that is both healing and nourishing.

Embracing dietary management as a cornerstone of diverticulitis care offers a path toward not just symptom relief but also long-term wellness. This chapter lays the groundwork for a deeper exploration of the condition, equipping you with the understanding necessary to navigate diverticulitis with confidence. Through a combination of diet, lifestyle adjustments, and medical care, you can reclaim control over your health and well-being.

As we advance to the next chapters, we'll delve into the practical aspects of managing diverticulitis, from symptom-specific recipes to strategies for meal planning and preparation, all designed to support you at every stage of your journey.

Chapter 2:   Navigating Your Diet Through the Stages of Diverticulitis

A Journey of Adaptation
Embarking on the journey of managing diverticulitis through dietary means is akin to learning a new language. This chapter is dedicated to translating the complex signals of your body into actionable insights, helping you navigate your diet through the different stages of diverticulitis. Understanding these stages is crucial in adopting a diet that not only addresses symptoms but also fosters long-term digestive health.

The Acute Phase: Crisis Management

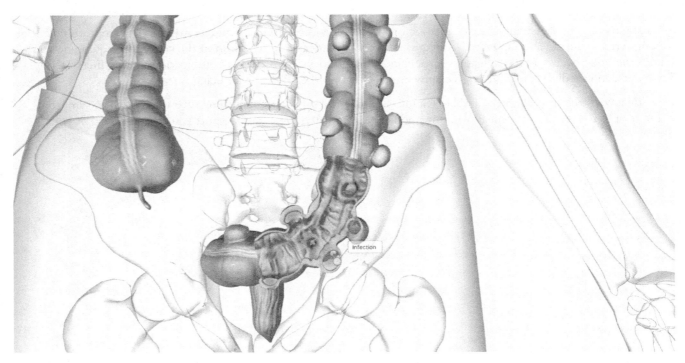

The acute phase represents the body's cry for a respite, a plea for healing from the intense turmoil of diverticulitis flare-ups. During this critical period, the dietary strategy leans heavily towards minimalism. The goal is to provide the body with necessary hydration and nutrients without taxing the already inflamed digestive system.

- **Liquid Nourishment**: The initiation of a clear liquid diet is akin to pressing a gentle pause on digestion, allowing the body to focus on healing. Broths, unsweetened teas, and clear juices become the mainstay, offering soothing hydration and vital electrolytes without stimulating further digestive activity. This approach serves a dual purpose: addressing immediate hydration needs while setting the stage for the digestive tract's recovery.
- **Gradual Introduction**: As the fiercest symptoms begin to wane, the diet cautiously evolves, introducing low-fiber foods that promise nourishment without adversity. Applesauce and cooked carrots epitomize this transition, providing vitamins and minerals in a form that's gentle on the gut. This phase is pivotal, marking the body's gradual readiness to accept more substantial nourishment. It's a deliberate, carefully monitored progression that underscores the healing journey, preparing the digestive system for a return to a semblance of normalcy.

The Recovery Phase: Building Strength
Post-crisis, the narrative shifts from immediate symptom management to fostering resilience within the digestive tract. This recovery phase is characterized by a strategic, mindful reintroduction of a broader spectrum of foods, each chosen for its potential to fortify and strengthen the gut without reigniting inflammation.

- **Fiber on the Horizon**: The reintroduction of fiber is approached with caution, starting with foods that offer a gentle reintroduction to this essential nutrient. The selection expands to include soft, cooked fruits and vegetables, and, in time, small portions of whole grains. Each addition is chosen for its digestibility and potential to contribute to the digestive tract's recovery, signaling a careful move towards a more fiber-rich diet that supports long-term gut health.
- **Listening to Your Body**: Central to this phase is the cultivation of a deep attunement to the body's signals. It's an exercise in patience and observation, recognizing that the path to recovery is not linear but undulating. Some days may welcome dietary exploration, while others necessitate a retreat to simpler fare. This responsiveness to the body's needs highlights the personalized nature of diverticulitis management, where flexibility and adaptation are paramount.

The Maintenance Phase: Prevention and Prosperity

In the maintenance phase, the focus pivots towards the future, laying the groundwork to minimize the risk of future flare-ups through a balanced, nutrient-rich diet.

- **Fiber-Full Diet**: A diversified, high-fiber diet becomes the cornerstone of this phase, embracing a wide array of fruits, vegetables, legumes, and whole grains. This dietetic approach not only aids in regularizing bowel movements but also in fortifying the colon walls, reducing the likelihood of diverticula formation and inflammation.
- **Hydration and Balance**: Hydration remains a crucial element, working in tandem with increased fiber intake to facilitate smooth, effortless bowel movements. The integration of varied food groups ensures a nutritional balance, supporting overall health without overburdening the digestive system. Meal timing and portion control also play vital roles, helping to maintain digestive equilibrium and supporting the body's natural healing and preventive mechanisms.

Navigating through these phases with a thoughtful, adaptable approach to diet can significantly impact the management of diverticulitis, promoting healing, strength, and long-term digestive wellness.

Tailoring Your Diet to Your Journey

Diverticulitis is a highly individual condition, and there's no one-size-fits-all diet. Use this chapter as a guide to understand the principles behind dietary management at each stage, but remember to customize these recommendations to fit your unique journey. Regular consultations with healthcare professionals can provide personalized advice, ensuring your diet aligns with your health needs and lifestyle.

Navigating your diet through the stages of diverticulitis empowers you to take control of your health. By understanding how to adapt your eating habits in response to your body's needs, you cultivate a supportive, healing relationship with food. This chapter aims to equip you with the knowledge and tools to manage your condition proactively, laying the foundation for a healthier, more vibrant life.

Part II: Recipes for Each Stage of Diverticulitis

Chapter 3: Acute Phase: Clear Liquid and Low-Fiber Recipes

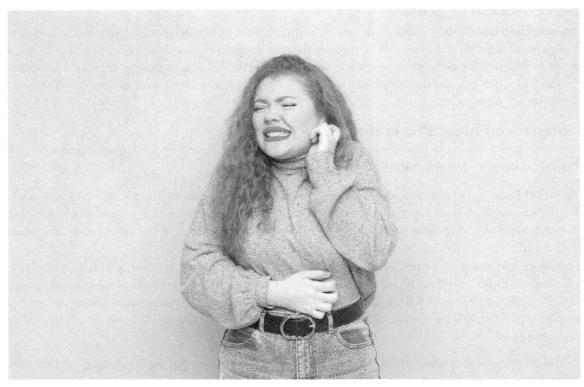

In the acute phase of diverticulitis, where inflammation is at its peak, the primary goal of your diet should be to minimize further irritation to your digestive tract and facilitate healing. This chapter of our cookbook is meticulously designed with this delicate balance in mind, offering a selection of recipes that cater specifically to the nutritional needs and limitations during this challenging time.

Understanding that your body requires ample rest and minimal digestive workload during a flare-up, the recipes in this chapter focus on liquid and very low-fiber foods. These meals are crafted to ensure you remain nourished and hydrated without exacerbating symptoms or delaying recovery.

- **Liquid Nutrition**: The acute phase recipes emphasize broths, herbal teas, and hydrating beverages that provide essential nutrients in the gentlest manner possible. These liquids help maintain hydration, a critical component of your body's healing process during a flare-up.
- **Ease and Simplicity**: Recognizing that your energy and appetite may be limited during this time, each recipe is designed to be straightforward and easy to prepare. From soothing clear broths to nourishing, smooth applesauce, the focus is on simplicity and comfort.
- **Foundational Foods for Gradual Transition**: As your symptoms begin to subside, this chapter also introduces very low-fiber foods that can serve as the foundation for your gradual transition back to a more varied diet. These include options like boiled potatoes (without the skin) and white rice, which provide energy without significant fiber content.

This chapter acts as a gentle guide for navigating the acute phase of diverticulitis, offering recipes that support healing and provide relief. By prioritizing liquid and very low-fiber foods, we aim to alleviate your symptoms while ensuring your body receives the nutrition it needs to recover. As always, we recommend consulting with your healthcare provider before making any dietary changes, especially during a diverticulitis flare-up, to ensure the choices you make are aligned with your current health needs and recovery process.

Breakfast Recipes

1. Gentle Ginger Tea

Prep Time: 5 minutes | **Cooking Time:** 10 minutes | **Serving Size:** 1 serving

Ingredients:
- 1-inch fresh ginger root, thinly sliced
- 1 cup water
- Honey or lemon juice to taste (optional)

Instructions:
1. In a small saucepan, bring the water and ginger slices to a boil. Lower the heat and let simmer for about 10 minutes to allow the ginger to infuse.
2. Strain the tea into a cup, removing the ginger slices.
3. Add honey or lemon juice to taste, if desired.
4. Serve the tea warm for soothing comfort.

Nutritional Information: Calories: <10 (without honey) | Carbs: 2g | Fat: 0g | Protein: 0g | Fibers: 0g

Tip: Ginger tea can help soothe the digestive system. Adjust the amount of ginger to suit your taste and tolerance, especially during the acute phase of diverticulitis.

2. Clear Chicken Broth

Prep Time: 5 minutes | **Cooking Time:** 25 minutes | **Serving Size:** 2 servings

Ingredients:
- 4 cups water
- 1 small chicken breast (bone-in for more flavor, optional)
- 1/2 teaspoon salt (optional, adjust based on dietary needs)
- 1 bay leaf (optional)
- A few slices of ginger (optional, for additional soothing properties)

Instructions:
1. Combine water, chicken breast, salt, bay leaf, and ginger slices in a large pot. Bring to a boil over high heat.
2. Once boiling, reduce the heat to a low simmer. Cover and let it cook for about 20-25 minutes, or until the chicken is fully cooked.
3. Carefully remove the chicken breast from the broth. You can shred it for later use in other recipes if desired.
4. Strain the broth through a fine mesh sieve to remove the bay leaf, ginger, and any solids.
5. Serve the broth warm, either as is for a soothing drink or use it as a base for other recipes.

Nutritional Information: Calories: 15 | Carbs: 0g | Fat: 0.5g | Protein: 2g | Fibers: 0g

Tip: This clear broth is perfect for the acute phase of diverticulitis when solid foods are best avoided. For additional flavor without added strain on the digestive system, consider simmering the broth with aromatic herbs like thyme or parsley stems, remembering to strain them out before serving.

3. Soothing Rice Porridge

Prep Time: 5 minutes | **Cooking Time:** 30 minutes | **Serving Size:** 2 servings

Ingredients:
- 1/2 cup white rice, rinsed
- 4 cups water or low-sodium chicken broth
- Pinch of salt (optional)

Instructions:
1. In a medium saucepan, combine the rinsed white rice and water (or broth) and bring to a boil over medium-high heat.
2. Once boiling, reduce the heat to low, cover, and simmer for about 30 minutes, or until the rice is very soft and the mixture has a porridge-like consistency.
3. Stir occasionally to prevent sticking and add more water if necessary to achieve the desired consistency.
4. Season with a pinch of salt if desired, and serve warm.

Nutritional Information: Calories: 120 | Carbs: 26g | Fat: 0g | Protein: 2g | Fibers: 1g

Tip: For a gentle flavor boost, you can add a slice of ginger to the cooking water, remembering to remove it before serving. This porridge is easily digestible and can be customized with tolerated toppings as you move further along in your recovery phase.

4. Basic Apple Gelatin

Prep Time: 10 minutes (plus chilling time) | **Cooking Time:** 5 minutes | **Serving Size:** 4 servings

Ingredients:
- 2 cups unsweetened apple juice, divided
- 2 tablespoons unflavored gelatin powder
- 1/2 teaspoon cinnamon (optional)
- Honey or maple syrup to taste (optional)

Instructions:
1. Pour 1/2 cup of apple juice into a small bowl. Sprinkle the gelatin powder over the juice and let it sit for about 5 minutes to soften.
2. Heat the remaining 1 1/2 cups of apple juice in a saucepan over medium heat until just starting to simmer. Do not boil.
3. Add the softened gelatin mixture to the hot apple juice, stirring until the gelatin is completely dissolved. Remove from heat.
4. Stir in cinnamon and honey or maple syrup if using, mixing well.
5. Pour the mixture into a shallow dish or individual molds. Refrigerate until set, about 3 hours.
6. Serve chilled, cut into squares or unmolded.

Nutritional Information: Calories: 100 | Carbs: 24g | Fat: 0g | Protein: 2g | Fibers: 0g

Tip: This apple gelatin can be a refreshing, easily digestible treat during the recovery phase. For an additional layer of flavor without adding solid pieces, consider infusing the apple juice with a bag of chamomile tea while heating, removing it before adding the gelatin.

5. Herbal Infusion Blend

Prep Time: 5 minutes | **Cooking Time:** 10 minutes | **Serving Size:** 2 servings

Ingredients:
- 2 cups boiling water
- 1 teaspoon chamomile flowers
- 1 teaspoon peppermint leaves
- 1 teaspoon lemon balm leaves
- Honey to taste (optional)

Instructions:
1. Boil 2 cups of water in a kettle.
2. Place chamomile, peppermint, and lemon balm leaves in a teapot or a heatproof container.
3. Pour the boiling water over the herbs and cover. Let steep for 10 minutes to allow the flavors and properties of the herbs to infuse into the water.
4. Strain the infusion into cups, discarding the used herbs.
5. Sweeten with honey if desired and serve warm.

Nutritional Information: Calories: <5 (without honey) | Carbs: 1g | Fat: 0g | Protein: 0g | Fibers: 0g

Tip: This herbal blend is designed to soothe and relax, making it perfect for evenings. Feel free to adjust the herb quantities to your taste or based on what's well tolerated during your phase of diverticulitis management.

6. Plain Rice Water

Prep Time: 5 minutes | **Cooking Time:** 30 minutes | **Serving Size:** 2 servings

Ingredients:
- 1/2 cup white rice
- 4 cups water

Instructions:
1. Rinse the white rice under cold water until the water runs clear.
2. In a large pot, combine the rinsed rice and 4 cups of water. Bring to a boil over high heat.
3. Once boiling, reduce the heat to a simmer and cover. Let it cook for about 30 minutes.
4. Strain the mixture, collecting the water in a container. The rice can be saved for other uses or consumed separately if your dietary phase allows.
5. Serve the rice water warm, or allow it to cool and refrigerate for a chilled drink.

Nutritional Information: Calories: 0 | Carbs: 0g | Fat: 0g | Protein: 0g | Fibers: 0g

Tip: Rice water is known for its soothing properties on the digestive system. For a slight flavor enhancement without adding irritants, consider adding a dash of cinnamon or ginger to the water during the cooking process, ensuring to strain it out before drinking.

7. Low-Fiber Cream of Wheat

Prep Time: 5 minutes | **Cooking Time:** 10 minutes | **Serving Size:** 2 servings

Ingredients:
- 1/2 cup cream of wheat (uncooked)
- 2 cups water or milk (for a creamier texture)
- Pinch of salt
- Honey or maple syrup to taste (optional)

Instructions:
1. In a medium saucepan, bring the water or milk to a boil. Add a pinch of salt.
2. Gradually whisk in the cream of wheat, ensuring there are no lumps.
3. Reduce the heat to low and simmer, stirring frequently, for about 10 minutes, or until the mixture thickens to your liking.
4. Remove from heat and let it stand for a couple of minutes to cool slightly. The cream of wheat will continue to thicken as it cools.
5. Sweeten with honey or maple syrup if desired, and serve warm.

Nutritional Information: Calories: 150 | Carbs: 32g | Fat: 0g | Protein: 4g | Fibers: 1g

Tip: For an easily digestible breakfast or snack during the recovery phase, cream of wheat can be a comforting option. Its smooth texture is gentle on the digestive system, and you can adjust the thickness by adding more or less liquid.

8. Simple Poached Pear

Prep Time: 5 minutes | **Cooking Time:** 25 minutes | **Serving Size:** 2 servings

Ingredients:
- 2 ripe pears, peeled
- 4 cups water
- 1 cinnamon stick (optional)
- 2 cloves (optional)
- 1 star anise (optional)
- Honey or maple syrup for drizzling (optional)

Instructions:
1. In a large saucepan, bring the water to a simmer over medium heat. If using, add the cinnamon stick, cloves, and star anise to the water for flavor.
2. Carefully place the peeled pears into the simmering water. Reduce heat to low and cover.
3. Poach the pears for about 20-25 minutes, or until they are tender when pierced with a fork.
4. Gently remove the pears from the water and let them cool slightly.
5. Serve the pears warm or chilled, with a drizzle of honey or maple syrup if desired.

Nutritional Information: Calories: 100 | Carbs: 27g | Fat: 0g | Protein: 0g | Fibers: 5g

Tip: Poached pears are a gentle, fiber-rich dessert option perfect for the recovery phase. The spices can be adjusted or omitted based on your tolerance and preferences. This simple yet elegant dish can be a soothing end to a meal.

9. Bland Scrambled Egg Whites

Prep Time: 2 minutes | **Cooking Time:** 5 minutes | **Serving Size:** 1 serving

Ingredients:
- 3 egg whites
- 1 tablespoon water
- Salt to taste

Instructions:
1. In a small bowl, whisk together the egg whites, water, and a pinch of salt until well combined.
2. Heat a non-stick skillet over medium heat and lightly coat it with cooking spray or a small amount of oil.
3. Pour the egg mixture into the skillet and let it cook for about 1-2 minutes, or until the edges begin to set.
4. Using a spatula, gently push the cooked edges towards the center of the skillet, allowing the uncooked eggs to flow to the edges.
5. Continue cooking and gently stirring the eggs until they are fully cooked but still moist, about 2-3 minutes more.
6. Remove the skillet from heat and transfer the scrambled egg whites to a plate.
7. Serve immediately, plain or with a sprinkle of salt if desired.

Nutritional Information: Calories: 51 | Carbs: 0g | Fat: 0g | Protein: 11g | Fibers: 0g

Tip: These bland scrambled egg whites are gentle on the digestive system, making them suitable for the acute phase of diverticulitis. Customize them by adding herbs or spices as tolerated during the recovery and maintenance phases.

10. Steamed White Rice Mash

Prep Time: 2 minutes | **Cooking Time:** 20 minutes | **Serving Size:** 2 servings

Ingredients:
- 1 cup white rice
- 2 cups water

Instructions:
1. Rinse the white rice under cold water until the water runs clear.
2. In a medium saucepan, combine the rinsed rice and water.
3. Bring the water to a boil over medium-high heat.
4. Once boiling, reduce the heat to low and cover the saucepan with a tight-fitting lid.
5. Simmer the rice for 15-20 minutes, or until all the water is absorbed and the rice is tender.
6. Remove the saucepan from heat and let it sit, covered, for an additional 5 minutes to allow the rice to steam.
7. Fluff the rice with a fork and mash it lightly with the back of a spoon to achieve a softer texture.
8. Serve the steamed white rice mash warm as a gentle side dish.

Nutritional Information: Calories: 110 | Carbs: 24g | Fat: 0g | Protein: 2g | Fibers: 0g

Tip: This simple steamed white rice mash provides a bland yet comforting option for those in the acute phase of diverticulitis. Customize it by adding a pat of butter or a sprinkle of salt for extra flavor during the recovery and maintenance phases.

Snack Recipes

11. Soothing Clear Broth Cubes

Prep Time: 5 minutes | **Cooking Time:** 5 minutes | **Servings:** 4

Ingredients:

- 4 cups of low-sodium chicken or vegetable broth

Instructions:

1. **Prepare the Broth:** In a medium saucepan, bring the low-sodium chicken or vegetable broth to a gentle boil.
2. **Pour and Freeze:** Carefully pour the broth into an ice cube tray and let it cool. Place the tray in the freezer and freeze until the broth cubes are solid, about 2-3 hours.
3. **Serve:** To use, dissolve 1-2 broth cubes in a cup of hot water for a soothing drink.

Nutritional Information: Calories: 5 (per cube) | Carbs: 0g | Fat: 0g | Protein: 1g | Fibers: 0g

Tip: These broth cubes are a convenient way to ensure you can quickly prepare a soothing, warm broth, especially beneficial during the acute phase of diverticulitis for easy digestion and hydration.

12. Gentle Apple and Cinnamon Compote

Prep Time: 5 minutes | **Cooking Time:** 15 minutes | **Servings:** 2

Ingredients:

- 2 large apples, peeled, cored, and sliced
- 1/2 cup water
- 1/4 teaspoon ground cinnamon
- 1 teaspoon honey or maple syrup (optional)

Instructions:

1. **Combine Ingredients:** In a saucepan over medium heat, combine the apple slices, water, and cinnamon. Stir gently to mix.
2. **Cook:** Cover the saucepan and let the mixture simmer for about 15 minutes, or until the apples are soft and tender. Stir occasionally to prevent sticking.
3. **Mash:** Once the apples are fully softened, remove from heat. You can mash the apples with a fork or potato masher for a smoother texture. Stir in honey or maple syrup if desired for additional sweetness.
4. **Serve:** Allow the compote to cool slightly before serving. It can be enjoyed warm or cold.

Nutritional Information: Calories: 90 | Carbs: 24g | Fat: 0g | Protein: 0g | Fibers: 4g

Tip: This apple and cinnamon compote is ideal for the acute phase of diverticulitis as it's gentle on the digestive system while providing a comforting, naturally sweet snack. Serve it as is, or over a small portion of low-fiber custard for an extra treat.

13. Hydrating Herbal Ice Pops

Prep Time: 5 minutes + freezing time | **Cooking Time:** 0 minutes | **Servings:** 4

Ingredients:

- 2 cups of your favorite herbal tea, brewed and cooled (such as chamomile or peppermint)
- 1 tablespoon honey or maple syrup (optional, to taste)

Instructions:

1. **Sweeten the Tea:** Once your herbal tea has cooled to room temperature, stir in honey or maple syrup if using, until well dissolved.
2. **Pour into Molds:** Carefully pour the sweetened herbal tea into ice pop molds.
3. **Freeze:** Insert sticks into the molds. Place the molds in the freezer and freeze until solid, about 4-6 hours or overnight.
4. **Serve:** To release the ice pops, run warm water over the outside of the molds for a few seconds. Gently pull the sticks to remove the ice pops and enjoy a refreshing, hydrating treat.

Nutritional Information: Calories: 15 (per pop) | Carbs: 4g | Fat: 0g | Protein: 0g | Fibers: 0g

Tip: These herbal ice pops are perfect for staying hydrated during the acute phase of diverticulitis, offering a soothing and refreshing way to consume fluids without irritating the digestive system. Choose herbal teas that you find comforting and relaxing.

14. Cooling Peppermint Tea Gelatin

Prep Time: 5 minutes | **Cooking Time:** 5 minutes | **Setting Time:** 3 hours | **Servings:** 4

Ingredients:

- 2 cups peppermint tea, brewed strong
- 2 tablespoons honey or maple syrup (optional)
- 2 teaspoons unflavored gelatin powder

Instructions:

1. **Prepare the Tea:** Brew the peppermint tea and let it cool slightly. If desired, dissolve honey or maple syrup in the warm tea for a touch of sweetness.
2. **Bloom the Gelatin:** Sprinkle the gelatin powder over 1/2 cup of cold water in a small bowl. Let it sit for 1-2 minutes until the gelatin softens.
3. **Dissolve the Gelatin:** Heat the softened gelatin mixture over low heat, stirring constantly, until the gelatin dissolves completely. Do not boil.
4. **Combine:** Pour the dissolved gelatin into the brewed tea and stir well.
5. **Set:** Pour the mixture into molds or a shallow dish. Refrigerate until set, about 3 hours.
6. **Serve:** Once set, cut into cubes or shapes if using a shallow dish, or release from molds if used.

Nutritional Information: Calories: 30 | Carbs: 8g | Fat: 0g | Protein: 0g | Fibers: 0g

Tip: This cooling peppermint tea gelatin is a soothing snack perfect for the acute phase of diverticulitis. Peppermint is known for its digestive benefits, making this a great choice for easing symptoms while staying hydrated.

15. Simple Honey-Drizzled Poached Pears

Prep Time: 5 minutes | **Cooking Time:** 25 minutes | **Servings:** 2

Ingredients:

- 2 ripe pears, peeled, halved, and cored
- 4 cups of water
- 1 cinnamon stick
- 2 tablespoons honey

Instructions:

1. **Poach the Pears:** In a large saucepan, combine the water and cinnamon stick and bring to a simmer. Add the pear halves. Simmer gently for 20-25 minutes, or until the pears are tender when pierced with a fork.

2. **Serve:** Carefully remove the pear halves from the liquid and place them on serving dishes.

3. **Drizzle with Honey:** Drizzle each pear half with honey before serving.

Nutritional Information: Calories: 120 | Carbs: 32g | Fat: 0g | Protein: 0g | Fibers: 5g

Tip: These simple honey-drizzled poached pears are a sweet and gentle treat suitable for the acute phase of diverticulitis. The soft texture of the pears makes them easy to digest, while the honey adds a natural sweetness without the need for refined sugars.

Lunch Recipes

16. Broth-Based Vegetable Soup

Prep Time: 10 minutes | **Cooking Time:** 25 minutes | **Serving Size:** 4 servings

Ingredients:

- 4 cups low-sodium chicken broth
- 1 cup diced carrots
- 1 cup diced celery
- 1 cup diced zucchini
- 1 cup diced potatoes
- Salt and pepper to taste
- Chopped fresh parsley for garnish (optional)

Instructions:

1. In a large pot, bring the low-sodium chicken broth to a boil over medium-high heat.
2. Add the diced carrots, celery, zucchini, and potatoes to the pot.
3. Reduce the heat to low and let the soup simmer for 20-25 minutes, or until the vegetables are tender.
4. Season the soup with salt and pepper to taste.
5. Ladle the broth-based vegetable soup into bowls and garnish with chopped fresh parsley if desired.
6. Serve hot and enjoy!

Nutritional Information: Calories: 70 | Carbs: 14g | Fat: 0g | Protein: 3g | Fibers: 2g

Tip: This broth-based vegetable soup is gentle on the digestive system and provides essential nutrients during the acute phase of diverticulitis. Customize it by adding other soft vegetables as tolerated.

17. Mashed Carrot Puree

Prep Time: 5 minutes | **Cooking Time:** 20 minutes | **Serving Size:** 2 servings

Ingredients:

- 2 cups diced carrots
- 1 cup low-sodium chicken broth
- Salt to taste
- Fresh parsley for garnish (optional)

Instructions:

1. In a medium saucepan, combine the diced carrots and low-sodium chicken broth.
2. Bring the mixture to a boil over medium-high heat.
3. Reduce the heat to low, cover the saucepan, and let the carrots simmer for 15-20 minutes, or until they are very tender.
4. Using a slotted spoon, transfer the cooked carrots to a blender or food processor, reserving the cooking liquid.

5. Blend the carrots until smooth, adding small amounts of the reserved cooking liquid as needed to achieve your desired consistency.

6. Season the mashed carrot puree with salt to taste.

7. Transfer the puree to a serving dish and garnish with fresh parsley if desired.

8. Serve warm as a comforting side dish.

Nutritional Information: Calories: 70 | Carbs: 16g | Fat: 0g | Protein: 2g | Fibers: 4g

Tip: This mashed carrot puree is easy to digest and provides a boost of vitamin A and fiber. Customize it by adding a pinch of ground ginger or cinnamon for extra flavor.

18. Tender Chicken Broth Soup

Prep Time: 5 minutes | **Cooking Time:** 25 minutes | **Serving Size:** 4 servings

Ingredients:
- 4 cups low-sodium chicken broth
- 1 cup diced cooked chicken breast
- 1 cup diced carrots
- 1 cup diced celery
- Salt and pepper to taste
- Chopped fresh parsley for garnish (optional)

Instructions:
1. In a large pot, bring the low-sodium chicken broth to a boil over medium-high heat.
2. Add the diced cooked chicken breast, carrots, and celery to the pot.
3. Reduce the heat to low and let the soup simmer for 20-25 minutes, or until the vegetables are tender.
4. Season the soup with salt and pepper to taste.
5. Ladle the tender chicken broth soup into bowls and garnish with chopped fresh parsley if desired.
6. Serve hot and enjoy!

Nutritional Information: Calories: 90 | Carbs: 5g | Fat: 1g | Protein: 15g | Fibers: 1g

Tip: This tender chicken broth soup is gentle on the digestive system and provides a comforting source of protein. Customize it by adding other soft vegetables or herbs as tolerated.

19. Soft-Cooked Acorn Squash

Prep Time: 5 minutes | **Cooking Time:** 30 minutes | **Serving Size:** 2 servings

Ingredients:

- 1 acorn squash
- 1 tablespoon olive oil
- Salt and pepper to taste

Instructions:

1. Preheat your oven to 400°F (200°C).
2. Using a sharp knife, carefully cut the acorn squash in half lengthwise and scoop out the seeds and stringy pulp.
3. Place the squash halves, cut-side up, on a baking sheet lined with parchment paper.
4. Drizzle the olive oil over the squash halves and season with salt and pepper to taste.
5. Roast the squash in the preheated oven for 25-30 minutes, or until the flesh is soft and fork-tender.
6. Remove the squash from the oven and let it cool slightly before serving.
7. Using a spoon, scoop out the soft flesh of the acorn squash and transfer it to a serving dish.
8. Serve the soft-cooked acorn squash warm as a nutritious side dish.

Nutritional Information: Calories: 120 | Carbs: 20g | Fat: 5g | Protein: 2g | Fibers: 4g

Tip: This soft-cooked acorn squash is rich in vitamins and minerals, making it a nourishing option during the acute phase of diverticulitis. Customize it by sprinkling with cinnamon or nutmeg for added flavor.

20. Plain Gelatin Cups

Prep Time: 5 minutes | **Cooking Time:** 5 minutes, plus chilling time | **Serving Size:** 4 servings

Ingredients:

- 2 packets unflavored gelatin
- 2 cups water
- Fresh fruit slices for garnish (optional)

Instructions:

1. In a small saucepan, sprinkle the unflavored gelatin evenly over the water and let it sit for 2-3 minutes to soften.
2. Place the saucepan over low heat and stir continuously until the gelatin has completely dissolved, about 2-3 minutes.
3. Remove the saucepan from the heat and pour the gelatin mixture into individual serving cups or molds.
4. Let the gelatin cups cool to room temperature, then cover them with plastic wrap and refrigerate for at least 2-3 hours, or until set.
5. Once set, remove the gelatin cups from the refrigerator and garnish with fresh fruit slices if desired.
6. Serve the plain gelatin cups chilled as a light and refreshing dessert option.

Nutritional Information: Calories: 5 | Carbs: 0g | Fat: 0g | Protein: 1g | Fibers: 0g

Tip: These plain gelatin cups are easy to digest and provide a simple, low-calorie treat during the acute phase of diverticulitis. Customize them by using fruit-flavored gelatin or adding chopped fruit before chilling.

21. Silky Potato Soup

Prep Time: 10 minutes | **Cooking Time:** 25 minutes | **Serving Size:** 4 servings

Ingredients:
- 2 tablespoons unsalted butter
- 1 onion, diced
- 2 cloves garlic, minced
- 4 cups low-sodium chicken broth
- 4 cups peeled and diced potatoes
- Salt and pepper to taste
- 1/2 cup heavy cream
- Chopped chives for garnish (optional)

Instructions:
1. In a large pot, melt the unsalted butter over medium heat.
2. Add the diced onion and minced garlic to the pot and cook until softened, about 5 minutes.
3. Pour the low-sodium chicken broth into the pot and add the diced potatoes.
4. Bring the mixture to a boil, then reduce the heat to low and let it simmer for 15-20 minutes, or until the potatoes are tender.
5. Using an immersion blender or regular blender, puree the soup until smooth.
6. Stir in the heavy cream and season the soup with salt and pepper to taste.
7. Continue to cook the soup for another 5 minutes, or until heated through.
8. Ladle the silky potato soup into bowls and garnish with chopped chives if desired.
9. Serve hot and enjoy this comforting and nourishing dish!

Nutritional Information: Calories: 250 | Carbs: 30g | Fat: 12g | Protein: 5g | Fibers: 3g

Tip: This silky potato soup is gentle on the stomach and provides a creamy texture without the need for high-fiber ingredients. Customize it by adding shredded cheese or bacon bits for extra flavor.

22. Low-Fiber Baked Apple

Prep Time: 5 minutes | **Cooking Time:** 30 minutes | **Serving Size:** 2 servings

Ingredients:
- 2 apples (such as Fuji or Gala)
- 1 tablespoon unsalted butter
- 1 tablespoon honey
- 1/2 teaspoon ground cinnamon
- 1/4 cup water

Instructions:
1. Preheat your oven to 375°F (190°C).

2. Wash and core the apples, removing the seeds and stems.

3. Place the cored apples in a baking dish.

4. In a small bowl, mix together the unsalted butter, honey, and ground cinnamon.

5. Stuff each cored apple with the butter-honey mixture.

6. Pour the water into the bottom of the baking dish.

7. Cover the baking dish with aluminum foil and bake the apples in the preheated oven for 20 minutes.

8. Remove the foil and continue baking for another 10 minutes, or until the apples are soft and tender.

9. Serve the low-fiber baked apples warm, optionally topped with a dollop of Greek yogurt or a sprinkle of chopped nuts.

Nutritional Information: Calories: 140 | Carbs: 30g | Fat: 4g | Protein: 1g | Fibers: 5g

Tip: These low-fiber baked apples are a delicious and comforting dessert option during the acute phase of diverticulitis. Customize them by using different spices such as nutmeg or cloves for added flavor.

23. Clear Beef Broth

Prep Time: 5 minutes | **Cooking Time:** 2 hours | **Serving Size:** 4 servings

Ingredients:
- 1 pound beef bones (such as marrow bones or soup bones)
- 8 cups water
- Salt to taste

Instructions:
1. Rinse the beef bones under cold water to remove any debris or impurities.

2. Place the beef bones in a large pot and cover them with water.

3. Bring the water to a boil over high heat, then reduce the heat to low and let the broth simmer gently.

4. Skim off any foam or impurities that rise to the surface of the broth with a spoon.

5. Let the broth simmer uncovered for 1.5 to 2 hours, allowing the flavors to develop and the broth to reduce.

6. Remove the pot from the heat and strain the broth through a fine-mesh sieve or cheesecloth to remove any bone fragments or sediment.

7. Season the clear beef broth with salt to taste, if desired.

8. Serve the clear beef broth hot as a comforting and nourishing beverage, or use it as a base for soups and other dishes.

Nutritional Information: Calories: 0 | Carbs: 0g | Fat: 0g | Protein: 0g | Fibers: 0g

Tip: This clear beef broth is gentle on the stomach and provides essential hydration and nourishment during the acute phase of diverticulitis. Customize it by adding herbs and spices such as bay leaves, peppercorns, or thyme for extra flavor.

24. Simple Poached Chicken Breast

Prep Time: 5 minutes | **Cooking Time:** 20 minutes | **Serving Size:** 2 servings

Ingredients:
- 2 boneless, skinless chicken breasts
- 4 cups low-sodium chicken broth or water
- Salt and pepper to taste

Instructions:
1. In a medium-sized pot, bring the low-sodium chicken broth or water to a gentle simmer over medium heat.
2. Season the chicken breasts with salt and pepper to taste.
3. Carefully add the seasoned chicken breasts to the simmering liquid, ensuring they are fully submerged.
4. Cover the pot with a lid and let the chicken breasts poach in the liquid for 15-20 minutes, or until they are cooked through and no longer pink in the center.
5. Use tongs to remove the poached chicken breasts from the liquid and transfer them to a cutting board.
6. Allow the chicken breasts to rest for a few minutes before slicing them thinly against the grain.
7. Serve the simple poached chicken breast slices warm alongside steamed vegetables or a light salad for a nutritious and satisfying meal.

Nutritional Information: Calories: 170 | Carbs: 0g | Fat: 3g | Protein: 32g | Fibers: 0g

Tip: This simple poached chicken breast recipe is a gentle and versatile option during the acute phase of diverticulitis. Customize it by adding herbs and aromatics such as garlic, onion, or thyme to the poaching liquid for extra flavor.

25. Pureed Pumpkin Soup

Prep Time: 10 minutes | **Cooking Time:** 30 minutes | **Serving Size:** 4 servings

Ingredients:
- 1 tablespoon olive oil
- 1 small onion, chopped
- 2 cloves garlic, minced
- 1 medium-sized pumpkin, peeled, seeded, and cubed
- 4 cups low-sodium chicken or vegetable broth
- Salt and pepper to taste
- Optional garnish: chopped fresh parsley or a dollop of Greek yogurt

Instructions:
1. In a large pot, heat the olive oil over medium heat. Add the chopped onion and minced garlic, and sauté until softened and fragrant, about 3-5 minutes.
2. Add the cubed pumpkin to the pot and sauté for another 5 minutes, stirring occasionally.

3. Pour the low-sodium chicken or vegetable broth into the pot, ensuring the pumpkin is fully submerged. Bring the mixture to a boil, then reduce the heat to low and let it simmer, covered, for 20-25 minutes, or until the pumpkin is tender.

4. Use an immersion blender or transfer the soup to a blender in batches to puree until smooth.

5. Season the pureed pumpkin soup with salt and pepper to taste, adjusting the seasoning as needed.

6. Ladle the soup into bowls and garnish with chopped fresh parsley or a dollop of Greek yogurt, if desired.

7. Serve the pureed pumpkin soup warm, alongside a slice of whole-grain bread or a light salad for a comforting meal.

Nutritional Information: Calories: 100 | Carbs: 15g | Fat: 4g | Protein: 2g | Fibers: 3g

Tip: This pureed pumpkin soup is a soothing and nutritious option during the acute phase of diverticulitis. Customize it by adding spices such as cinnamon, nutmeg, or ginger for extra warmth and flavor.

Dinner Recipes

26. Butternut Squash Puree

Prep Time: 15 minutes | **Cooking Time:** 30 minutes | **Serving Size:** 4 servings

Ingredients:

- 1 medium butternut squash, peeled, seeded, and diced
- 1 tablespoon olive oil
- 1 small onion, chopped
- 2 cloves garlic, minced
- 4 cups low-sodium vegetable broth
- Salt and pepper to taste
- Optional garnish: chopped fresh chives or a dollop of Greek yogurt

Instructions:

1. In a large pot, heat the olive oil over medium heat. Add the chopped onion and minced garlic, and sauté until softened and fragrant, about 3-5 minutes.
2. Add the diced butternut squash to the pot and sauté for another 5 minutes, stirring occasionally.
3. Pour the low-sodium vegetable broth into the pot, ensuring the butternut squash is fully submerged. Bring the mixture to a boil, then reduce the heat to low and let it simmer, covered, for 20-25 minutes, or until the butternut squash is tender.
4. Use an immersion blender or transfer the soup to a blender in batches to puree until smooth.
5. Season the butternut squash puree with salt and pepper to taste, adjusting the seasoning as needed.
6. Ladle the puree into bowls and garnish with chopped fresh chives or a dollop of Greek yogurt, if desired.
7. Serve the butternut squash puree warm, alongside a slice of whole-grain bread or a light salad for a comforting meal.

Nutritional Information: Calories: 120 | Carbs: 28g | Fat: 3g | Protein: 2g | Fibers: 6g

Tip: Butternut squash is rich in vitamins and minerals, making this puree not only soothing but also nutritious. Experiment with different herbs and spices to enhance the flavor, such as cinnamon, nutmeg, or sage.

27. Strained Lentil Soup

Prep Time: 10 minutes | **Cooking Time:** 40 minutes | **Serving Size:** 4 servings

Ingredients:

- 1 cup dried lentils, rinsed and drained
- 4 cups low-sodium vegetable broth
- 1 medium carrot, peeled and diced
- 1 stalk celery, diced
- 1 small onion, chopped
- 2 cloves garlic, minced
- 1 bay leaf
- Salt and pepper to taste

- Optional garnish: chopped fresh parsley or a drizzle of olive oil

Instructions:
1. In a large pot, combine the dried lentils, low-sodium vegetable broth, diced carrot, diced celery, chopped onion, minced garlic, and bay leaf.
2. Bring the mixture to a boil over medium-high heat, then reduce the heat to low and let it simmer, covered, for 30-35 minutes, or until the lentils are tender.
3. Once the lentils are cooked, remove the bay leaf from the pot and discard it.
4. Using an immersion blender or transferring the soup to a blender in batches, blend the soup until smooth.
5. If desired, strain the blended soup through a fine-mesh sieve or cheesecloth to remove any remaining fibrous bits and achieve a smoother texture.
6. Season the strained lentil soup with salt and pepper to taste, adjusting the seasoning as needed.
7. Ladle the soup into bowls and garnish with chopped fresh parsley or a drizzle of olive oil, if desired.
8. Serve the strained lentil soup warm, accompanied by a slice of crusty bread or a side salad for a satisfying meal.

Nutritional Information: Calories: 160 | Carbs: 28g | Fat: 1g | Protein: 12g | Fibers: 10g

Tip: Lentils are a great source of plant-based protein and fiber, making this soup not only comforting but also filling and nutritious. Feel free to customize the soup by adding additional vegetables or herbs to suit your taste preferences.

28. Steamed White Fish Fillet

Prep Time: 5 minutes | **Cooking Time:** 10 minutes | **Serving Size:** 2 servings

Ingredients:
- 2 white fish fillets (such as tilapia, cod, or haddock), about 4-6 ounces each
- 1 lemon, thinly sliced
- Salt and pepper to taste
- Fresh herbs for garnish (optional)

Instructions:
1. Season the white fish fillets with salt and pepper on both sides.
2. Place a steamer basket in a large pot filled with a couple of inches of water. Make sure the water level is below the bottom of the steamer basket.
3. Arrange the lemon slices in the steamer basket, creating a bed for the fish fillets to rest on.
4. Carefully place the seasoned fish fillets on top of the lemon slices in the steamer basket.
5. Cover the pot with a lid and bring the water to a boil over medium-high heat.
6. Once the water is boiling, reduce the heat to medium-low and let the fish steam for 8-10 minutes, or until it is opaque and flakes easily with a fork.
7. Remove the pot from the heat and carefully transfer the steamed fish fillets to serving plates.
8. Garnish the fish with fresh herbs, if desired, and serve immediately with a side of steamed vegetables or a light salad for a simple yet satisfying meal.

Nutritional Information: Calories: 120 | Carbs: 0g | Fat: 2g | Protein: 25g | Fibers: 0g

Tip: Steaming is a gentle cooking method that helps preserve the delicate flavor and texture of fish while keeping it moist and tender. Experiment with different herbs and seasonings to customize the flavor of the steamed white fish fillets to your liking.

29. Baked Sweet Potato Mash

Prep Time: 10 minutes | **Cooking Time:** 45 minutes | **Serving Size:** 4 servings

Ingredients:

- 2 large sweet potatoes, peeled and cubed
- 2 tablespoons olive oil
- 1 tablespoon honey (optional)
- Salt and pepper to taste
- Optional toppings: chopped fresh herbs, toasted nuts, or a drizzle of maple syrup

Instructions:

1. Preheat your oven to 400°F (200°C).
2. Place the cubed sweet potatoes on a baking sheet lined with parchment paper.
3. Drizzle the olive oil over the sweet potatoes and toss them to coat evenly.
4. Season the sweet potatoes with salt and pepper to taste, and drizzle with honey if using.
5. Spread the sweet potatoes out in a single layer on the baking sheet.
6. Roast the sweet potatoes in the preheated oven for 40-45 minutes, or until they are tender and caramelized, stirring halfway through cooking.
7. Once the sweet potatoes are cooked, remove them from the oven and transfer them to a mixing bowl.
8. Mash the roasted sweet potatoes with a fork or potato masher until smooth and creamy.
9. Taste the mashed sweet potatoes and adjust the seasoning if needed.
10. Serve the baked sweet potato mash warm, topped with your choice of chopped fresh herbs, toasted nuts, or a drizzle of maple syrup for added flavor and texture.

Nutritional Information: Calories: 180 | Carbs: 30g | Fat: 6g | Protein: 2g | Fibers: 4g

Tip: Sweet potatoes are naturally sweet and packed with fiber, vitamins, and minerals, making them a nutritious and delicious addition to your diet. Experiment with different seasonings and toppings to create unique flavor combinations for your baked sweet potato mash.

30. Clear Tomato Broth

Prep Time: 5 minutes | **Cooking Time:** 20 minutes | **Serving Size:** 4 servings

Ingredients:

- 4 cups water
- 2 large tomatoes, quartered
- 1 small onion, chopped
- 2 cloves garlic, minced
- 1 teaspoon olive oil
- Salt and pepper to taste
- Fresh basil leaves for garnish (optional)

Instructions:

1. In a large pot, heat the olive oil over medium heat.

2. Add the chopped onion and minced garlic to the pot and sauté until the onion is soft and translucent, about 3-4 minutes.

3. Add the quartered tomatoes to the pot and cook for another 5 minutes, stirring occasionally.

4. Pour the water into the pot and bring the mixture to a boil.

5. Once boiling, reduce the heat to low and let the broth simmer uncovered for 10-15 minutes, allowing the flavors to meld together.

6. Season the broth with salt and pepper to taste.

7. Remove the pot from the heat and strain the clear tomato broth through a fine mesh sieve or cheesecloth into a clean bowl, discarding the solids.

8. Divide the clear tomato broth among serving bowls and garnish with fresh basil leaves, if desired.

9. Serve the clear tomato broth hot as a comforting and soothing soup, or use it as a base for other recipes.

Nutritional Information: Calories: 20 | Carbs: 4g | Fat: 0g | Protein: 1g | Fibers: 1g

Tip: This clear tomato broth is light, refreshing, and packed with the natural sweetness of ripe tomatoes. Enjoy it as a nourishing and hydrating soup on its own, or use it as a flavorful base for risottos, stews, or pasta dishes.

31. Low-Fiber Turkey Soup

Prep Time: 15 minutes | **Cooking Time:** 1 hour | **Serving Size:** 6 servings

Ingredients:

- 1 lb (450g) boneless, skinless turkey breast, cubed
- 1 tablespoon olive oil
- 1 onion, diced
- 2 carrots, diced
- 2 celery stalks, diced
- 4 cups low-sodium chicken broth
- 2 cups water
- 1 bay leaf
- Salt and pepper to taste
- Chopped fresh parsley for garnish (optional)

Instructions:

1. In a large pot, heat the olive oil over medium heat.

2. Add the diced onion, carrots, and celery to the pot and sauté until the vegetables are soft, about 5-7 minutes.

3. Add the cubed turkey breast to the pot and cook until lightly browned on all sides, about 5 minutes.

4. Pour the low-sodium chicken broth and water into the pot, and add the bay leaf.

5. Bring the soup to a boil, then reduce the heat to low and let it simmer uncovered for 45 minutes to 1 hour, stirring occasionally.

6. Once the turkey is cooked through and the vegetables are tender, remove the pot from the heat.

7. Season the soup with salt and pepper to taste, and discard the bay leaf.

8. Ladle the low-fiber turkey soup into serving bowls, garnish with chopped fresh parsley if desired, and serve hot.

Nutritional Information: Calories: 150 | Carbs: 5g | Fat: 4g | Protein: 22g | Fibers: 1g

Tip: This low-fiber turkey soup is hearty, comforting, and perfect for soothing sore stomachs during diverticulitis flare-ups. Feel free to customize it with your favorite herbs and spices for extra flavor.

32. Gentle Zucchini Soup

Prep Time: 10 minutes | **Cooking Time:** 25 minutes | **Serving Size:** 4 servings

Ingredients:
- 2 medium zucchinis, diced
- 1 tablespoon olive oil
- 1 onion, diced
- 2 cloves garlic, minced
- 4 cups low-sodium vegetable broth
- 1 teaspoon dried thyme
- Salt and pepper to taste
- Fresh parsley for garnish (optional)

Instructions:
1. In a large pot, heat the olive oil over medium heat.

2. Add the diced onion and minced garlic to the pot and sauté until fragrant and translucent, about 3-4 minutes.

3. Add the diced zucchinis to the pot and cook for another 5 minutes, stirring occasionally.

4. Pour the low-sodium vegetable broth into the pot and bring the mixture to a boil.

5. Once boiling, reduce the heat to low and let the soup simmer uncovered for 15-20 minutes, allowing the flavors to meld together.

6. Stir in the dried thyme, and season the soup with salt and pepper to taste.

7. Remove the pot from the heat and let the soup cool slightly.

8. Use an immersion blender to puree the soup until smooth and creamy.

9. Ladle the gentle zucchini soup into serving bowls, garnish with fresh parsley if desired, and serve hot.

Nutritional Information: Calories: 70 | Carbs: 8g | Fat: 4g | Protein: 2g | Fibers: 2g

Tip: This gentle zucchini soup is light, nourishing, and easy on the digestive system. Feel free to adjust the seasoning and consistency to suit your preferences.

33. Plain Gelatin with Fruit Juice

Prep Time: 5 minutes | **Chilling Time:** 4 hours | **Serving Size:** 4 servings

Ingredients:
- 1 packet (0.25 oz) unflavored gelatin
- 1 cup fruit juice of your choice (e.g., apple, grape, or cranberry)

Instructions:
1. In a small saucepan, pour the fruit juice and sprinkle the unflavored gelatin evenly over the surface. Allow it to sit for 2-3 minutes to soften.
2. Place the saucepan over low heat and stir constantly until the gelatin is completely dissolved, about 2-3 minutes. Do not let the mixture boil.
3. Once the gelatin is fully dissolved, remove the saucepan from the heat and let the mixture cool slightly.
4. Pour the liquid gelatin into individual serving cups or molds.
5. Place the cups or molds in the refrigerator and let the gelatin set for at least 4 hours, or until firm.
6. Once set, remove the plain gelatin from the refrigerator and serve chilled.

Nutritional Information: Calories: 20 | Carbs: 5g | Fat: 0g | Protein: 1g | Fibers: 0g

Tip: This plain gelatin with fruit juice is a soothing and easy-to-digest treat during diverticulitis flare-ups. You can customize the flavor by using your favorite fruit juice, or even mix different juices for a unique taste experience.

34. Poached Cod in Broth

Prep Time: 10 minutes | **Cooking Time:** 15 minutes | **Serving Size:** 2 servings

Ingredients:
- 2 cod fillets (about 6 ounces each)
- 4 cups low-sodium vegetable broth
- 1 lemon, thinly sliced
- 2 cloves garlic, minced
- 1 teaspoon dried thyme
- Salt and pepper to taste
- Fresh parsley for garnish (optional)

Instructions:
1. In a large skillet or shallow pan, pour the low-sodium vegetable broth and add the thinly sliced lemon, minced garlic, and dried thyme.
2. Heat the broth over medium heat until it comes to a gentle simmer.
3. Season the cod fillets with salt and pepper to taste, then carefully place them in the simmering broth.
4. Let the cod fillets poach in the broth for about 10-12 minutes, or until they are opaque and flake easily with a fork.
5. Once cooked, carefully remove the poached cod fillets from the broth using a slotted spoon and transfer them to serving plates.
6. Ladle some of the warm broth over the cod fillets, garnish with fresh parsley if desired, and serve immediately.

Nutritional Information: Calories: 250 | Carbs: 6g | Fat: 2g | Protein: 50g | Fibers: 1g

Tip: This poached cod in broth is a gentle and flavorful dish that's easy on the digestive system. Serve it alongside steamed vegetables or a simple salad for a complete and nourishing meal.

35.   Smooth Carrot and Ginger Soup

Prep Time: 10 minutes | **Cooking Time:** 25 minutes | **Serving Size:** 4 servings

Ingredients:

- 1 tablespoon olive oil
- 1 onion, chopped
- 2 cloves garlic, minced
- 1 tablespoon fresh ginger, grated
- 4 cups low-sodium vegetable broth
- 1 pound carrots, peeled and chopped
- Salt and pepper to taste
- Fresh parsley for garnish (optional)

Instructions:

1. In a large pot, heat the olive oil over medium heat. Add the chopped onion and cook until translucent, about 5 minutes.
2. Add the minced garlic and grated ginger to the pot, and cook for an additional 2 minutes, until fragrant.
3. Pour the low-sodium vegetable broth into the pot, and add the chopped carrots. Bring the mixture to a boil, then reduce the heat and let it simmer for about 15-20 minutes, or until the carrots are tender.
4. Once the carrots are cooked through, use an immersion blender to puree the soup until smooth. Alternatively, you can transfer the soup in batches to a blender and blend until smooth.
5. Season the soup with salt and pepper to taste, and adjust the seasoning as needed.
6. Serve the smooth carrot and ginger soup hot, garnished with fresh parsley if desired.

Nutritional Information: Calories: 120 | Carbs: 18g | Fat: 4g | Protein: 2g | Fibers: 4g

Tip: This smooth carrot and ginger soup is a comforting and nourishing option during the recovery phase of diverticulitis. The combination of carrots and ginger provides both sweetness and warmth, while the smooth texture makes it easy to digest.

Chapter 4: Recovery Phase: Low to Moderate Fiber Recipes

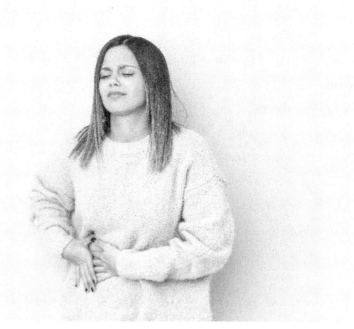

This chapter marks a significant transition in your journey with diverticulitis, focusing on the recovery phase—a period of gradual healing and reintroduction of a broader variety of foods into your diet. As your digestive system begins to recover from a flare-up, it's crucial to provide it with the nutrients needed for healing while still being mindful of its current sensitivities. This chapter offers a curated collection of recipes designed specifically for this delicate balance, aiding in your recovery and setting the foundation for long-term digestive health.

During the recovery phase, the dietary focus shifts from the very low-fiber, liquid-based diet of the acute phase to incorporating more substantial but still gentle foods. The recipes in this chapter are crafted with this transition in mind, featuring meals that are nourishing, easy to digest, and gradually reintroduce fiber to your diet in a manageable way.

- **Nutrient-Rich Soups**: Soups that are slightly more substantial than broths, enriched with pureed vegetables and tender proteins, provide essential vitamins and minerals without overwhelming your digestive system.
- **Soft-Cooked Vegetables**: Gentle on the gut, these recipes emphasize vegetables cooked until soft, making them easier to digest and providing necessary nutrients without excessive fiber.
- **Protein-Packed Dishes**: Lean proteins like chicken, fish, and tofu, prepared in simple, digestible ways, support tissue repair and overall health during recovery.
- **Gradual Fiber Introduction**: Carefully selected grains and legumes are introduced in modest amounts, helping your digestive system adjust to fiber more gradually.

Each recipe is accompanied by guidance on how to adjust fiber content and portion sizes to match your current stage of recovery and personal tolerance levels. This personalized approach ensures that you can enjoy a varied diet that supports your healing without risking a setback in your progress.

In navigating the recovery phase with the support of this chapter, you're taking an essential step towards not just managing diverticulitis, but thriving despite it. These recipes are your companions on the path to recovery, designed to bring joy back to eating while honoring the needs of your healing body.

Breakfast Recipes

36. Creamy Oatmeal with Mashed Banana

Prep Time: 5 minutes | **Cooking Time:** 10 minutes | **Servings:** 2

Ingredients:

- 1 cup rolled oats
- 2 cups water or milk
- 1 ripe banana, mashed
- 1/2 teaspoon vanilla extract
- 1 tablespoon honey or maple syrup (optional)
- A pinch of cinnamon
- A pinch of salt

Instructions:

1. **Prepare the Oats:** In a medium saucepan, bring the water or milk to a boil. Add the oats and a pinch of salt, then reduce the heat to a simmer.
2. **Cook:** Allow the oats to cook for 5-10 minutes, stirring occasionally, until they have absorbed the liquid and are fully cooked.
3. **Add Flavors:** Remove the saucepan from heat. Stir in the mashed banana, vanilla extract, and cinnamon. Add honey or maple syrup if desired.
4. **Serve:** Divide the oatmeal into bowls. If you like, sprinkle a little more cinnamon on top for garnish.

Nutritional Information: Calories: 220 | Carbs: 45g | Fat: 3g | Protein: 6g | Fibers: 5g

Tip: This oatmeal is perfect for the recovery phase, providing a nutritious, gentle introduction to fiber. The mashed banana adds natural sweetness and a creamy texture.

37. Scrambled Eggs with Avocado

Prep Time: 5 minutes | **Cooking Time:** 5 minutes | **Servings:** 2

Ingredients:

- 4 large eggs
- 1 ripe avocado, peeled and sliced
- 2 tablespoons milk (optional, for creamier eggs)
- Salt and pepper to taste
- 1 tablespoon olive oil or butter

Instructions:

1. **Beat the Eggs:** In a bowl, whisk together the eggs, milk (if using), salt, and pepper until well combined and slightly frothy.

2. **Cook the Eggs:** Heat the olive oil or butter in a non-stick skillet over medium heat. Pour in the egg mixture. Let it sit, without stirring, for a few seconds until the eggs start to set around the edges.

3. **Scramble:** With a spatula, gently stir the eggs, pushing from the edges towards the center. Cook until the eggs are softly set and slightly runny in places, about 3-4 minutes. Remove from heat as they will continue to cook in the pan.

4. **Serve with Avocado:** Divide the scrambled eggs onto plates and top with sliced avocado. Season with additional salt and pepper to taste.

Nutritional Information: Calories: 290 | Carbs: 9g | Fat: 23g | Protein: 13g | Fibers: 7g

Tip: This dish offers a balanced mix of healthy fats, protein, and fiber, ideal for the recovery phase of diverticulitis. Avocado not only adds creaminess and flavor but also provides beneficial monounsaturated fats.

38. Baked Pears with Honey

Prep Time: 5 minutes | **Cooking Time:** 25 minutes | **Servings:** 2

Ingredients:

- 2 ripe pears, halved and cored

- 2 teaspoons honey

- A pinch of ground cinnamon

- 1/4 cup water

Instructions:

1. **Prepare the Pears:** Preheat your oven to 350°F (175°C). Arrange the pear halves, cut-side up, in a baking dish. Drizzle each pear half evenly with honey and then sprinkle with a pinch of cinnamon.

2. **Bake:** Pour the water into the bottom of the baking dish around the pear halves. This will help to keep the pears moist as they bake. Bake in the preheated oven for 25 minutes, or until the pears are tender and cooked through.

3. **Serve:** Allow the pears to cool slightly before serving. They can be enjoyed warm or at room temperature.

Nutritional Information: Calories: 110 | Carbs: 29g | Fat: 0g | Protein: 1g | Fibers: 5g

Tip: Baked pears with honey offer a sweet treat without overwhelming your digestive system during the recovery phase. The natural sweetness of the pears makes this a comforting dessert or snack.

39. Cottage Cheese with Soft Peaches

Prep Time: 5 minutes | **No Cooking Required** | **Servings:** 2

Ingredients:

- 1 cup low-fat cottage cheese
- 1 ripe peach, peeled and sliced
- 1 teaspoon honey (optional)
- A pinch of ground cinnamon (optional)

Instructions:

1. **Prepare the Peach:** Peel the peach and cut it into thin slices. If peaches are not in season, canned peaches in natural juice (well-drained) can also be a convenient and tasty alternative.
2. **Assemble the Dish:** Divide the cottage cheese between two bowls. Top each bowl with half of the sliced peaches. Drizzle with honey and sprinkle a pinch of cinnamon over the top, if desired.
3. **Serve:** Enjoy this dish as a refreshing and nutritious breakfast or snack. It's ready to eat with no cooking required.

Nutritional Information: Calories: 150 | Carbs: 15g | Fat: 2g | Protein: 14g | Fibers: 1g

Tip: This simple yet nutritious recipe combines the creamy texture of cottage cheese with the sweet, soft texture of peaches, offering a gentle way to include protein and fruit in your diet during the recovery phase. Adjust the sweetness to your liking with honey and add a hint of cinnamon for an extra flavor dimension.

40. Smooth Peanut Butter on Toasted White Bread

Prep Time: 2 minutes | **Cooking Time:** 3 minutes | **Servings:** 2

Ingredients:

- 4 slices white bread, preferably low-fiber
- 4 tablespoons smooth peanut butter
- 1 banana, thinly sliced (optional)
- A drizzle of honey (optional)

Instructions:

1. **Toast the Bread:** Lightly toast the slices of white bread until they are just golden and slightly crispy.
2. **Spread Peanut Butter:** Spread 1 tablespoon of smooth peanut butter evenly over each slice of toasted bread.
3. **Add Toppings:** If using, place banana slices on top of the peanut butter for added sweetness and texture. Drizzle with a little honey for extra flavor if desired.
4. **Serve:** Cut each slice into halves or quarters for easier eating and serve immediately.

Nutritional Information: Calories: 290 | Carbs: 34g | Fat: 16g | Protein: 10g | Fibers: 3g

Tip: This easy and satisfying recipe provides a good balance of protein and carbohydrates. Smooth peanut butter and white bread are chosen for their gentleness on the digestive system during the recovery phase. The optional banana adds natural sweetness and soft texture that's also easy to digest.

41. Rice Porridge with Maple Syrup

Prep Time: 5 minutes | **Cooking Time:** 25 minutes | **Servings:** 2

Ingredients:

- 1/2 cup white rice, rinsed
- 2 cups water or milk for a creamier texture
- A pinch of salt
- 2 tablespoons maple syrup, or to taste
- A dash of cinnamon (optional)

Instructions:

1. **Cook the Rice:** In a medium saucepan, combine the rinsed white rice, water (or milk), and a pinch of salt. Bring to a boil over medium-high heat. Once boiling, reduce the heat to low, cover, and simmer for 20-25 minutes, or until the rice is tender and the liquid is mostly absorbed.
2. **Make the Porridge:** Remove the saucepan from the heat and let it stand covered for 5 minutes. The rice will continue to absorb any remaining liquid and become more porridge-like in consistency.
3. **Flavor the Porridge:** Stir in the maple syrup, adjusting the amount to your liking. Add a dash of cinnamon for a hint of spice, if desired.
4. **Serve:** Divide the rice porridge into bowls. Drizzle with a little more maple syrup and sprinkle with cinnamon if you used it in the recipe.

Nutritional Information: Calories: 210 | Carbs: 46g | Fat: 1g | Protein: 4g | Fibers: 1g

Tip: Rice porridge is a comforting and easily digestible option perfect for the recovery phase. The simple flavors of maple syrup and optional cinnamon make it a warm and satisfying breakfast or snack. For those advancing in their recovery, consider adding a small portion of sliced bananas or berries for added vitamins and gentle fiber.

42. Mashed Pumpkin Pancakes

Prep Time: 10 minutes | **Cooking Time:** 15 minutes | **Servings:** 2-3

Ingredients:

- 1 cup mashed pumpkin (canned pumpkin puree or fresh pumpkin that has been cooked and mashed)
- 1 cup all-purpose flour
- 2 teaspoons baking powder
- 1/2 teaspoon cinnamon (optional)
- A pinch of salt
- 1 egg, beaten
- 1 cup milk
- 2 tablespoons unsalted butter, melted, plus extra for cooking
- 2 tablespoons maple syrup, plus extra for serving

Instructions:

1. **Mix Dry Ingredients:** In a large bowl, combine the flour, baking powder, cinnamon (if using), and salt.

2. **Combine Wet Ingredients:** In another bowl, mix together the mashed pumpkin, beaten egg, milk, melted butter, and maple syrup until well combined.

3. **Make the Batter:** Gradually add the wet ingredients to the dry ingredients, stirring just until the batter is smooth and there are no lumps. Avoid overmixing.

4. **Cook the Pancakes:** Heat a non-stick skillet or griddle over medium heat and brush with a small amount of butter. Pour 1/4 cup of batter for each pancake onto the skillet. Cook until bubbles form on the surface, then flip and cook until golden brown on the other side, about 2-3 minutes per side.

5. **Serve:** Serve the pancakes warm, drizzled with additional maple syrup.

Nutritional Information: Calories: 260 | Carbs: 45g | Fat: 6g | Protein: 8g | Fibers: 2g

Tip: These pancakes offer a flavorful way to incorporate vegetables into your breakfast, providing vitamins and a hint of sweetness from the pumpkin. The texture is soft and easily digestible, making them a great option for the recovery phase. Adjust the amount of cinnamon and maple syrup to suit your taste and dietary needs.

43. Soft-Boiled Eggs with Saltine Crackers

Prep Time: 2 minutes | **Cooking Time:** 6 minutes | **Servings:** 2

Ingredients:

- 4 large eggs
- 8 saltine crackers
- Salt and pepper to taste

Instructions:

1. **Boil the Eggs:** Place the eggs in a saucepan and cover with cold water by an inch. Bring to a boil over medium-high heat. Once boiling, reduce the heat to low and simmer for about 5-6 minutes for soft-boiled eggs.

2. **Prepare the Eggs:** Remove the eggs from the heat, drain the hot water, and run cold water over the eggs to stop the cooking process. Once cool enough to handle, gently peel the eggs.

3. **Serve:** Place two soft-boiled eggs on each plate. Season with salt and pepper to taste. Serve with four saltine crackers on the side for each serving.

Nutritional Information: Calories: 170 | Carbs: 10g | Fat: 10g | Protein: 12g | Fibers: 0g

Tip: This simple yet nutritious meal is ideal for the recovery phase, providing easy-to-digest protein and a gentle texture. The saltine crackers offer a bland, comforting crunch that pairs well with the soft eggs. Adjust the cooking time if you prefer your eggs more or less runny.

44. Low-Fiber Blueberry Muffins

Prep Time: 10 minutes | **Cooking Time:** 20 minutes | **Servings:** 12 muffins

Ingredients:

- 2 cups all-purpose flour
- 1/2 cup sugar
- 3 teaspoons baking powder
- 1/2 teaspoon salt

- 3/4 cup milk
- 1/3 cup vegetable oil
- 1 egg
- 1 teaspoon vanilla extract
- 1 cup fresh blueberries (if in recovery phase, ensure they're well tolerated)

Instructions:

1. **Preheat Oven:** Preheat your oven to 400°F (200°C). Line a muffin tin with paper liners or lightly grease the tin.
2. **Combine Dry Ingredients:** In a large bowl, mix together the flour, sugar, baking powder, and salt.
3. **Mix Wet Ingredients:** In another bowl, beat together the milk, vegetable oil, egg, and vanilla extract until well combined.
4. **Combine Mixtures:** Add the wet ingredients to the dry ingredients, stirring just until the flour mixture is moistened. Do not overmix; the batter should be slightly lumpy.
5. **Add Blueberries:** Gently fold the blueberries into the batter, being careful not to crush them.
6. **Bake:** Spoon the batter into the prepared muffin tin, filling each cup about two-thirds full. Bake for 20 minutes, or until a toothpick inserted into the center of a muffin comes out clean.
7. **Cool:** Remove the muffins from the oven and allow them to cool in the pan for a few minutes before transferring them to a wire rack to cool completely.

Nutritional Information: Calories: 180 | Carbs: 28g | Fat: 6g | Protein: 3g | Fibers: 1g

Tip: These muffins offer a way to enjoy a sweet treat while keeping fiber content in check. For those in the recovery phase, start with a small portion to ensure it's well tolerated. These muffins can be frozen for later use, ensuring you have a quick, low-fiber option on hand.

45. Applesauce with Cinnamon Yogurt

Prep Time: 5 minutes | **No Cooking Required** | **Servings:** 2

Ingredients:

- 1 cup unsweetened applesauce
- 1/2 cup low-fat Greek yogurt
- 1/2 teaspoon ground cinnamon
- 1 teaspoon honey (optional)

Instructions:

1. **Mix the Yogurt:** In a small bowl, combine the Greek yogurt with ground cinnamon. Add honey to sweeten, if desired, and stir until well mixed.
2. **Assemble the Dish:** Spoon the unsweetened applesauce into two serving bowls.
3. **Add Yogurt:** Top each bowl of applesauce with half of the cinnamon yogurt mixture.
4. **Serve:** Enjoy immediately, or refrigerate for a chilled treat.

Nutritional Information: Calories: 120 | Carbs: 22g | Fat: 1g | Protein: 6g | Fibers: 2g

Tip: This simple, soothing recipe combines the natural sweetness of apples with the creamy tanginess of Greek yogurt, enhanced by the warm spice of cinnamon. It's an easy-to-prepare, comforting snack or dessert that's ideal for the recovery phase of diverticulitis, providing probiotics from the yogurt and a soft texture from the applesauce.

Snack Recipes

46. Mild Avocado Mash on Toasted White Bread

Prep Time: 5 minutes | **Cooking Time:** 2 minutes | **Servings:** 2

Ingredients:

- 1 ripe avocado
- 2 slices of white bread, toasted
- Pinch of salt
- Pinch of pepper (optional)

Instructions:

1. **Prepare the Avocado:** Cut the avocado in half, remove the pit, and scoop the flesh into a bowl. Mash the avocado with a fork until it reaches your desired consistency. Season with a pinch of salt and, if desired, a pinch of pepper.
2. **Toast the Bread:** While preparing the avocado, toast the white bread slices to your preference.
3. **Assemble:** Spread the mashed avocado evenly over the toasted white bread slices.
4. **Serve:** Enjoy the mild avocado mash on toast immediately for the freshest taste.

Nutritional Information: Calories: 230 | Carbs: 27g | Fat: 12g | Protein: 4g | Fibers: 7g

Tip: This snack is ideal for the recovery phase of diverticulitis, offering a soft, nutritious option that's gentle on the digestive system. The mild flavors of avocado and toast provide a comforting, easy-to-digest snack.

47. Baked Banana with a Dash of Cinnamon

Prep Time: 5 minutes | **Cooking Time:** 15 minutes | **Servings:** 2

Ingredients:

- 2 ripe bananas
- 1/2 teaspoon cinnamon

Instructions:

1. **Preheat Oven:** Preheat your oven to 350°F (175°C).
2. **Prepare Bananas:** Without peeling, slice the bananas lengthwise just deep enough to open them up a bit, but not all the way through. Sprinkle the inside of each banana with cinnamon.
3. **Bake:** Place the bananas on a baking sheet, cut side up, and bake in the preheated oven for about 15 minutes, or until the bananas are soft and the flavors have melded together.
4. **Serve:** Allow the bananas to cool slightly, then peel and enjoy warm for a cozy, naturally sweet snack.

Nutritional Information: Calories: 105 | Carbs: 27g | Fat: 0g | Protein: 1g | Fibers: 3g

Tip: This baked banana snack is perfect for the recovery phase, as it provides a warm, comforting option with a touch of cinnamon to aid digestion. It's a simple, wholesome way to satisfy a sweet craving without stressing the digestive system.

48. Creamy Low-Fiber Pumpkin Smoothie

Prep Time: 5 minutes | **Cooking Time:** 0 minutes | **Servings:** 2

Ingredients:

- 1/2 cup canned pumpkin puree (ensure it's plain pumpkin, not pie filling)
- 1 cup almond milk or any low-fat milk of your choice
- 1 banana
- 1/2 teaspoon vanilla extract
- 1/2 teaspoon pumpkin pie spice (optional)
- Ice cubes

Instructions:

1. **Blend Ingredients:** In a blender, combine the pumpkin puree, almond milk, banana, vanilla extract, and pumpkin pie spice if using. Add a handful of ice cubes.
2. **Puree until Smooth:** Blend on high speed until all ingredients are well combined and the mixture is smooth.
3. **Serve:** Pour the smoothie into glasses and serve immediately for a refreshing and creamy treat.

Nutritional Information: Calories: 120 | Carbs: 25g | Fat: 2g | Protein: 2g | Fibers: 3g

Tip: This smoothie is ideal for the recovery phase, providing a gently sweet and creamy option that's low in fiber yet satisfying. The pumpkin adds a dose of seasonal flavor and a smooth texture, making it a comforting choice for easing back into more diverse foods.

49. Soft-Cooked Apple and Pear Sauce

Prep Time: 10 minutes | **Cooking Time:** 20 minutes | **Servings:** 4

Ingredients:

- 2 apples, peeled, cored, and chopped
- 2 pears, peeled, cored, and chopped
- 1/2 cup water
- 1/4 teaspoon ground cinnamon
- 1 tablespoon honey or maple syrup (optional)

Instructions:

1. **Cook the Fruit:** In a large pot, combine the chopped apples, pears, water, and cinnamon. Bring to a simmer over medium heat, then cover and reduce the heat to low.
2. **Simmer:** Let the fruit simmer gently for about 20 minutes, or until it is completely soft and the flavors have melded.
3. **Mash:** Use a potato masher or fork to mash the cooked fruit to your desired consistency. For a smoother sauce, you can use a blender or food processor.
4. **Sweeten:** Stir in honey or maple syrup if using, adjusting the amount to taste.
5. **Serve:** Enjoy the apple and pear sauce warm, or allow it to cool and refrigerate before serving.

Nutritional Information: Calories: 110 | Carbs: 29g | Fat: 0g | Protein: 0g | Fibers: 5g

Tip: This comforting snack is perfect for the recovery phase, offering a naturally sweet treat that's easy on the digestive system. The soft texture and familiar flavors of apple and pear make this sauce a soothing choice for those easing back into a more varied diet.

50. Low-Fiber Berry and Yogurt Parfait

Prep Time: 5 minutes | **Cooking Time:** 0 minutes | **Servings:** 2

Ingredients:

- 1 cup low-fat Greek yogurt
- 1/2 cup mixed berries (such as strawberries and blueberries), chopped if large
- 1 tablespoon honey or maple syrup (optional)
- A sprinkle of ground cinnamon (optional)

Instructions:

1. **Layer the Parfait:** Begin by placing a layer of Greek yogurt at the bottom of two glasses or parfait dishes.
2. **Add Berries:** Add a layer of mixed berries over the yogurt.
3. **Repeat Layers:** Continue layering yogurt and berries until the glasses are filled, finishing with a layer of berries on top.
4. **Sweeten:** Drizzle honey or maple syrup over the top layer of berries, if desired.
5. **Garnish:** Sprinkle a little ground cinnamon over the berries for added flavor, if using.
6. **Serve:** Enjoy the parfait immediately for the freshest taste.

Nutritional Information: Calories: 150 | Carbs: 22g | Fat: 2g | Protein: 10g | Fibers: 2g

Tip: This berry and yogurt parfait is a delightful snack for the recovery phase, combining the creaminess of Greek yogurt with the fresh sweetness of berries. It's a visually appealing, nutritious option that's gentle on the digestive system while providing a boost of protein.

Lunch Recipes

51. Quinoa Salad with Roasted Vegetables

Prep Time: 15 minutes | **Cooking Time:** 25 minutes | **Servings:** 2

Ingredients:

- 1/2 cup quinoa, rinsed
- 1 cup water
- 1 small zucchini, diced
- 1 red bell pepper, diced
- 1/2 red onion, diced
- 2 tablespoons olive oil
- Salt and pepper to taste
- 2 tablespoons balsamic vinegar
- 1/4 cup feta cheese, crumbled (optional)
- Fresh basil leaves for garnish (optional)

Instructions:

1. **Cook Quinoa:** In a medium saucepan, bring 1 cup of water to a boil. Add the rinsed quinoa and a pinch of salt, then reduce the heat to low. Cover and simmer for 15 minutes, or until the water is absorbed and the quinoa is tender. Fluff with a fork and set aside to cool.

2. **Roast Vegetables:** Preheat your oven to 425°F (220°C). Toss the zucchini, bell pepper, and red onion with olive oil, salt, and pepper on a baking sheet. Roast for 20-25 minutes, stirring halfway through, until vegetables are tender and slightly caramelized.

3. **Assemble Salad:** In a large bowl, combine the cooked quinoa with the roasted vegetables. Drizzle with balsamic vinegar and toss to combine. Adjust seasoning with salt and pepper as needed.

4. **Serve:** Divide the salad between two plates. Top with crumbled feta cheese and garnish with fresh basil leaves if using.

Nutritional Information: Calories: 320 | Carbs: 45g | Fat: 12g | Protein: 10g | Fibers: 5g

Tip: This nutritious salad combines the hearty, nutty flavor of quinoa with the sweetness of roasted vegetables, offering a satisfying yet gentle meal suitable for the recovery phase. The feta cheese adds a tangy contrast, but can be omitted for a dairy-free version.

52. Baked Sweet Potato with Cottage Cheese

Prep Time: 5 minutes | **Cooking Time:** 45 minutes | **Servings:** 2

Ingredients:

- 2 medium sweet potatoes
- 1/2 cup low-fat cottage cheese
- Salt and pepper to taste
- A pinch of cinnamon (optional)
- Fresh chives, finely chopped for garnish (optional)

Instructions:

1. **Preheat Oven:** Preheat your oven to 400°F (200°C). Pierce the sweet potatoes several times with a fork to allow steam to escape during baking.
2. **Bake Sweet Potatoes:** Place the sweet potatoes on a baking sheet and bake in the preheated oven for 45 minutes, or until they are tender and fully cooked.
3. **Prepare Cottage Cheese:** While the sweet potatoes are baking, season the cottage cheese with salt and pepper. Add a pinch of cinnamon if desired, and stir to combine.
4. **Assemble:** Once the sweet potatoes are done, slice them open lengthwise, being careful not to cut all the way through. Fluff the insides with a fork.
5. **Serve:** Top each sweet potato with half of the seasoned cottage cheese. Garnish with chopped chives if using.

Nutritional Information: Calories: 250 | Carbs: 38g | Fat: 2g | Protein: 12g | Fibers: 5g

Tip: This recipe offers a nutritious, filling meal with a good balance of complex carbohydrates, protein, and a hint of sweetness from the cinnamon. The cottage cheese provides a creamy texture and protein boost, making it an excellent choice for those in the recovery phase looking for satisfying, gentle meals.

53. Pureed Butternut Squash Soup

Prep Time: 10 minutes | **Cooking Time:** 30 minutes | **Servings:** 2

Ingredients:

- 1 medium butternut squash, peeled, seeded, and cubed (about 2 cups)
- 1 tablespoon olive oil
- 1 small onion, chopped
- 2 cloves garlic, minced
- 3 cups vegetable broth
- Salt and pepper to taste
- 1/4 teaspoon ground nutmeg (optional)
- 2 tablespoons Greek yogurt for garnish (optional)
- Fresh parsley, chopped for garnish (optional)

Instructions:

1. **Sauté Vegetables:** In a large pot, heat the olive oil over medium heat. Add the chopped onion and garlic, sautéing until soft and translucent, about 5 minutes.

2. **Cook Squash:** Add the cubed butternut squash to the pot along with the vegetable broth. Bring to a boil, then reduce heat to low, cover, and simmer for about 20 minutes or until the squash is tender.

3. **Puree Soup:** Use an immersion blender to puree the soup directly in the pot until smooth. Alternatively, carefully transfer the soup to a blender, working in batches if necessary, and blend until smooth. Return the soup to the pot if using a standard blender.

4. **Season:** Add salt, pepper, and ground nutmeg to the soup, adjusting the seasonings to your taste. Heat through.

5. **Serve:** Ladle the soup into bowls. Garnish each serving with a dollop of Greek yogurt and a sprinkle of fresh parsley if desired.

Nutritional Information: Calories: 180 | Carbs: 30g | Fat: 5g | Protein: 4g | Fibers: 5g

Tip: This creamy butternut squash soup is naturally sweet, comforting, and packed with vitamins. It's easily digestible and the smooth texture makes it perfect for the recovery phase of diverticulitis. The Greek yogurt garnish adds a touch of creaminess and a boost of protein.

54. Soft-Cooked Chicken and Rice Bowl

Prep Time: 5 minutes | **Cooking Time:** 25 minutes | **Servings:** 2

Ingredients:

- 2 boneless, skinless chicken breasts
- 1 cup white rice, rinsed
- 2 cups low-sodium chicken broth
- Salt and pepper to taste
- 1/2 teaspoon dried thyme (optional)
- Fresh parsley, finely chopped for garnish (optional)

Instructions:

1. **Cook the Chicken:** In a medium saucepan, bring 1 cup of low-sodium chicken broth to a simmer. Add the chicken breasts, ensuring they are fully submerged. Cover and simmer over low heat for about 20 minutes, or until the chicken is cooked through and no longer pink inside. Remove the chicken, let it cool slightly, then shred or cut into bite-sized pieces.

2. **Cook the Rice:** In another saucepan, combine the rinsed white rice, the remaining 1 cup of chicken broth, and a pinch of salt. Bring to a boil, then reduce the heat to low, cover, and simmer for 18-20 minutes, or until the rice is tender and the liquid is absorbed.

3. **Assemble the Bowl:** Divide the cooked rice between two bowls. Top each bowl with half of the cooked chicken. Season with salt, pepper, and dried thyme, if using.

4. **Garnish and Serve:** Garnish with chopped fresh parsley before serving, if desired.

Nutritional Information: Calories: 350 | Carbs: 45g | Fat: 3g | Protein: 35g | Fibers: 1g

Tip: This simple, comforting chicken and rice bowl is easy to digest, making it a great choice for the recovery phase of diverticulitis. The dish is high in protein and provides a gentle way to reintroduce solid foods into your diet. Adjust the seasonings according to your taste and dietary tolerance.

55. Steamed Salmon with Mashed Cauliflower

Prep Time: 10 minutes | **Cooking Time:** 20 minutes | **Servings:** 2

Ingredients:

- 2 salmon fillets (about 6 ounces each)
- 1 medium head of cauliflower, cut into florets
- 2 tablespoons olive oil
- Salt and pepper to taste
- 1 tablespoon fresh lemon juice
- Fresh dill for garnish (optional)

Instructions:

1. **Steam the Salmon:** Fill a pot with a couple of inches of water and bring to a simmer. Place the salmon fillets in a steamer basket above the water, ensuring the water does not touch the fish. Cover and steam for about 10-12 minutes, or until the salmon is cooked through and flakes easily with a fork.
2. **Cook the Cauliflower:** While the salmon is steaming, place the cauliflower florets in a separate pot with about an inch of water. Cover and bring to a boil, then reduce heat and simmer for 10-15 minutes, or until the cauliflower is very tender.
3. **Mash the Cauliflower:** Drain the cauliflower well and return it to the pot. Add the olive oil, and mash the cauliflower with a potato masher or blend with an immersion blender until smooth. Season with salt and pepper to taste.
4. **Season the Salmon:** Once cooked, transfer the salmon to a plate and drizzle with fresh lemon juice. Add salt and pepper to taste.
5. **Serve:** Divide the mashed cauliflower onto plates, and place a salmon fillet on top of each. Garnish with fresh dill if using.

Nutritional Information: Calories: 390 | Carbs: 14g | Fat: 25g | Protein: 34g | Fibers: 5g

Tip: This meal combines the heart-healthy omega-3 fatty acids of salmon with the comforting texture of mashed cauliflower, making it ideal for those in the recovery phase seeking nutritious, easy-to-digest meals. The lemon juice adds a refreshing zing that complements the fish perfectly.

56. Turkey and Avocado Wrap with Soft Tortilla

Prep Time: 10 minutes | **No Cooking Required** | **Servings:** 2

Ingredients:

- 2 large soft tortillas (white flour recommended for lower fiber content)
- 6 ounces sliced turkey breast (deli style)
- 1 ripe avocado, mashed
- Salt and pepper to taste
- 1/4 cup shredded lettuce (optional, ensure it's tolerated)
- 2 tablespoons mayonnaise or Greek yogurt

Instructions:

1. **Prepare the Wraps:** Lay out the tortillas on a flat surface. Spread the mashed avocado evenly across each tortilla. Season with a little salt and pepper.
2. **Add Turkey:** Layer the sliced turkey breast on top of the mashed avocado on each tortilla. If using, add a thin layer of shredded lettuce over the turkey.
3. **Add Mayo or Yogurt:** Spread a tablespoon of mayonnaise or Greek yogurt over the turkey. This adds moisture and flavor to the wrap.
4. **Assemble:** Carefully roll up the tortillas tightly around the fillings. If necessary, you can secure the wraps with a toothpick.
5. **Serve:** Cut each wrap in half and serve immediately. For a softer eating experience, you can lightly grill the wraps on a panini press or skillet to warm them up without making them crispy.

Nutritional Information: Calories: 320 | Carbs: 27g | Fat: 16g | Protein: 20g | Fibers: 5g

Tip: This wrap is a great option for a nutritious and satisfying lunch that's easy on the digestive system during the recovery phase. The creamy texture of avocado and the lean protein from turkey make it both filling and gentle. Adjust the fillings based on your dietary needs and tolerances.

57. Low-Fiber Vegetable Stir-Fry with Tofu

Prep Time: 10 minutes | **Cooking Time:** 15 minutes | **Servings:** 2

Ingredients:

- 1/2 block firm tofu, pressed and cut into cubes
- 1 tablespoon olive oil
- 1/2 cup sliced bell peppers (red or yellow for milder flavor)
- 1/2 cup sliced carrots, thinly sliced
- 1/2 cup snap peas, strings removed (optional, ensure they're tolerated)
- 2 tablespoons low-sodium soy sauce or tamari
- 1 teaspoon sesame oil
- 1/2 teaspoon ground ginger
- Salt and pepper to taste

Instructions:

1. **Prepare Tofu:** Heat olive oil in a large non-stick skillet or wok over medium-high heat. Add the tofu cubes and fry until golden brown on all sides, about 5-7 minutes. Remove tofu from the skillet and set aside.
2. **Stir-Fry Vegetables:** In the same skillet, add a little more olive oil if needed. Stir-fry the bell peppers, carrots, and snap peas (if using) over high heat until just tender but still crisp, about 5-8 minutes.
3. **Combine Tofu and Vegetables:** Return the tofu to the skillet with the vegetables. Lower the heat to medium.
4. **Season:** Add the soy sauce, sesame oil, and ground ginger to the skillet. Toss well to combine and coat the tofu and vegetables evenly. Season with salt and pepper to taste.
5. **Serve:** Divide the stir-fry between two plates and serve immediately.

Nutritional Information: Calories: 220 | Carbs: 15g | Fat: 14g | Protein: 12g | Fibers: 3g

Tip: This vegetable stir-fry offers a nutritious meal with a good balance of protein from tofu and a variety of vegetables. It's designed to be low in fiber for those in the recovery phase, but always ensure the vegetables used are tolerated in your diet. The dish is flavorful and easy to digest, making it a satisfying meal option.

58. Pumpkin Soup with a Dollop of Greek Yogurt

Prep Time: 10 minutes | **Cooking Time:** 30 minutes | **Servings:** 2

Ingredients:

- 2 cups pumpkin puree (canned or fresh)
- 1 tablespoon olive oil
- 1 small onion, finely chopped
- 2 cloves garlic, minced
- 3 cups vegetable broth
- Salt and pepper to taste
- 1/4 teaspoon ground nutmeg (optional)
- 1/4 cup Greek yogurt for serving
- Fresh parsley or chives, chopped for garnish (optional)

Instructions:

1. **Sauté Onion and Garlic:** In a large pot, heat the olive oil over medium heat. Add the chopped onion and garlic, sautéing until soft and translucent, about 5 minutes.
2. **Cook Pumpkin:** Add the pumpkin puree to the pot along with the vegetable broth. Stir to combine. Bring to a boil, then reduce the heat to low and simmer for about 20-25 minutes, allowing the flavors to meld.
3. **Blend Soup:** Use an immersion blender to puree the soup directly in the pot until smooth. Alternatively, transfer the soup to a blender, working in batches if necessary, and blend until smooth. Return the soup to the pot if using a standard blender.
4. **Season:** Add salt, pepper, and ground nutmeg to the soup, adjusting the seasonings to your taste. Heat through.
5. **Serve:** Ladle the soup into bowls. Add a dollop of Greek yogurt to each serving and gently swirl with a spoon. Garnish with chopped parsley or chives if desired.

Nutritional Information: Calories: 180 | Carbs: 25g | Fat: 7g | Protein: 6g | Fibers: 6g

Tip: This comforting pumpkin soup is perfect for the recovery phase, offering a creamy texture and rich flavor without being too heavy. The Greek yogurt adds a nice tang and a boost of protein, making this dish both nutritious and satisfying. Adjust the thickness of the soup by adding more or less broth according to your preference.

59. Soft-Cooked Pasta with Olive Oil and Parmesan

Prep Time: 5 minutes | **Cooking Time:** 10 minutes | **Servings:** 2

Ingredients:

- 8 ounces pasta (choose a variety that is easy to digest, such as penne or fusilli)
- 2 tablespoons olive oil
- 1/4 cup grated Parmesan cheese
- Salt to taste
- Ground black pepper to taste (optional)
- Fresh basil leaves, torn for garnish (optional)

Instructions:

1. **Cook Pasta:** Bring a large pot of salted water to a boil. Add the pasta and cook according to package instructions until it is just tender but still firm to the bite (al dente). For a softer texture, which may be more suitable during the recovery phase, cook the pasta for an additional 1-2 minutes.
2. **Drain:** Once the pasta is cooked to your liking, drain it and return it to the pot or transfer it to a large bowl.
3. **Add Olive Oil and Cheese:** While the pasta is still hot, add the olive oil and grated Parmesan cheese. Toss until the pasta is evenly coated. Season with salt and, if using, ground black pepper to taste.
4. **Serve:** Divide the pasta between two serving dishes. Garnish with fresh basil leaves if desired.

Nutritional Information: Calories: 420 | Carbs: 56g | Fat: 16g | Protein: 16g | Fibers: 3g

Tip: This simple yet delicious pasta dish is perfect for those in the recovery phase looking for a meal that's easy on the stomach. The olive oil provides healthy fats, while the Parmesan adds a flavorful, cheesy depth. For an even gentler option, you can opt for pasta made from white flour rather than whole wheat or other grains with higher fiber content.

60. Lentil Stew with Carrots and Celery

Prep Time: 10 minutes | **Cooking Time:** 35 minutes | **Servings:** 2

Ingredients:

- 1 cup red lentils, rinsed and drained
- 4 cups low-sodium vegetable broth
- 1 medium carrot, peeled and diced
- 1 stalk celery, diced
- 1 small onion, finely chopped
- 2 cloves garlic, minced
- 1 tablespoon olive oil
- 1/2 teaspoon ground turmeric (optional)
- 1/2 teaspoon ground cumin (optional)
- Salt and pepper to taste

- Fresh parsley, chopped for garnish (optional)

Instructions:

1. **Sauté Vegetables:** In a large pot, heat the olive oil over medium heat. Add the onion, garlic, carrot, and celery. Sauté until the vegetables are softened, about 5 minutes.

2. **Cook Lentils:** Add the rinsed red lentils to the pot along with the vegetable broth. Stir in the ground turmeric and cumin if using. Bring the mixture to a boil, then reduce the heat to low. Cover and simmer for 25-30 minutes, or until the lentils are tender and the stew has thickened.

3. **Season:** Once the lentils are cooked, remove the pot from the heat. Season the stew with salt and pepper to taste.

4. **Serve:** Ladle the stew into bowls. Garnish with chopped parsley if desired.

Nutritional Information: Calories: 330 | Carbs: 55g | Fat: 7g | Protein: 18g | Fibers: 15g

Tip: This nutritious lentil stew is packed with protein and fiber, making it a hearty and comforting meal. The carrots and celery add a natural sweetness and texture to the dish. If you're in the recovery phase and concerned about fiber content, you can adjust the portion size or modify the amount of lentils to suit your dietary needs.

Dinner Recipes

61. Grilled Tilapia with Lemon Herb Dressing

Prep Time: 10 minutes | **Cooking Time:** 10 minutes | **Servings:** 2

Ingredients:

- 2 tilapia fillets (about 6 ounces each)
- 2 tablespoons olive oil
- Salt and pepper to taste
- 1 lemon, juiced and zested
- 1 tablespoon fresh parsley, finely chopped
- 1 tablespoon fresh dill, finely chopped
- 1 clove garlic, minced

Instructions:

1. **Preheat Grill:** Preheat your grill or grill pan over medium-high heat. Brush the grill grates with a little oil to prevent sticking.
2. **Prepare Tilapia:** Pat the tilapia fillets dry with paper towels. Brush both sides of the fillets with 1 tablespoon of olive oil and season with salt and pepper.
3. **Grill Tilapia:** Place the tilapia on the grill. Cook for about 4-5 minutes per side, or until the fish flakes easily with a fork and has nice grill marks.
4. **Make Lemon Herb Dressing:** In a small bowl, whisk together the remaining olive oil, lemon juice, lemon zest, parsley, dill, and minced garlic. Season with salt and pepper to taste.
5. **Serve:** Place the grilled tilapia on plates and drizzle with the lemon herb dressing. Serve immediately.

Nutritional Information: Calories: 280 | Carbs: 2g | Fat: 18g | Protein: 28g | Fibers: 0.5g

Tip: This light and flavorful dish is perfect for a recovery phase dinner, offering high-quality protein from the tilapia and a boost of fresh flavors from the lemon herb dressing. The dressing can be adjusted according to taste preferences or dietary needs.

62. Roasted Carrot and Ginger Soup

Prep Time: 15 minutes | **Cooking Time:** 45 minutes | **Servings:** 2

Ingredients:

- 1 pound carrots, peeled and chopped
- 1 tablespoon olive oil
- Salt and pepper to taste
- 2 cups vegetable broth
- 1 inch piece ginger, peeled and minced
- 1 small onion, chopped
- 1 clove garlic, minced
- 1/2 cup coconut milk
- Fresh parsley or cilantro, for garnish (optional)

Instructions:

1. **Roast Carrots:** Preheat your oven to 400°F (200°C). Toss the chopped carrots with olive oil, salt, and pepper on a baking sheet. Roast in the oven for 30-35 minutes, or until carrots are tender and slightly caramelized, stirring halfway through.

2. **Sauté Aromatics:** While the carrots are roasting, heat a teaspoon of olive oil in a large pot over medium heat. Add the chopped onion and minced ginger, cooking until the onion is translucent and soft, about 5 minutes. Add the garlic and cook for another minute until fragrant.

3. **Simmer Soup:** Add the roasted carrots to the pot with the vegetable broth. Bring to a simmer and cook for 10 minutes to allow the flavors to meld. Remove from heat and let cool slightly.

4. **Blend Soup:** Use an immersion blender to puree the soup directly in the pot until smooth. Alternatively, carefully transfer the soup to a blender, working in batches if necessary, and blend until smooth. Return the blended soup to the pot.

5. **Finish Soup:** Stir in the coconut milk and reheat the soup gently, making sure not to boil. Season with additional salt and pepper to taste.

6. **Serve:** Ladle the soup into bowls and garnish with fresh parsley or cilantro if desired.

Nutritional Information: Calories: 250 | Carbs: 30g | Fat: 14g | Protein: 3g | Fibers: 8g

Tip: This creamy, comforting soup pairs the sweet, earthy flavor of carrots with the warm spice of ginger, making it perfect for a cozy recovery phase meal. The coconut milk adds a rich creaminess without dairy, suitable for those with lactose intolerance or dairy restrictions.

63. Baked Cod with Soft Herbed Polenta

Prep Time: 10 minutes | **Cooking Time:** 25 minutes | **Servings:** 2

Ingredients:

- 2 cod fillets (about 6 ounces each)
- 1 tablespoon olive oil
- Salt and pepper to taste
- 1 lemon, sliced for garnish
- **For the Polenta:**
    - 1/2 cup polenta (cornmeal)
    - 2 cups water or low-sodium chicken broth
    - 1 tablespoon unsalted butter
    - 1/4 cup grated Parmesan cheese
    - 1 tablespoon fresh herbs (such as parsley or chives), chopped
    - Salt to taste

Instructions:

1. **Preheat Oven:** Preheat your oven to 375°F (190°C). Lightly oil a baking dish.
2. **Prepare Cod:** Place the cod fillets in the prepared baking dish. Brush each fillet with olive oil and season with salt and pepper. Arrange lemon slices around the fillets.
3. **Bake Cod:** Bake in the preheated oven for about 15-20 minutes, or until the fish flakes easily with a fork.
4. **Cook Polenta:** While the cod is baking, bring the water or chicken broth to a boil in a saucepan. Gradually whisk in the polenta, reducing the heat to low. Cook, stirring frequently, for about 15 minutes, or until the polenta is thick and creamy. Stir in the butter, Parmesan cheese, and fresh herbs. Season with salt to taste.
5. **Serve:** Spoon a generous amount of herbed polenta onto each plate. Place a baked cod fillet on top of the polenta. Garnish with additional fresh herbs and lemon slices from the baking dish.

Nutritional Information: Calories: 390 | Carbs: 35g | Fat: 16g | Protein: 35g | Fibers: 4g

Tip: This dish offers a balanced meal with lean protein from the cod and comforting, creamy polenta flavored with fresh herbs and Parmesan. It's a satisfying yet gentle option suitable for the recovery phase, with the soft textures making it easy on the digestive system.

64. Turkey Meatballs in Low-Fiber Tomato Sauce

Prep Time: 15 minutes | **Cooking Time:** 30 minutes | **Servings:** 2

Ingredients:

- **For the Turkey Meatballs:**
    - 1/2 pound ground turkey
    - 1/4 cup breadcrumbs (use low-fiber or gluten-free if needed)
    - 1 egg, beaten

- 1 tablespoon grated Parmesan cheese
- 1 teaspoon dried oregano
- Salt and pepper to taste
- **For the Sauce:**
  - 1 tablespoon olive oil
  - 1 small onion, finely chopped
  - 2 cloves garlic, minced
  - 1 can (14 oz) low-fiber tomato sauce (look for no added seeds or skins)
  - Salt and pepper to taste
  - Fresh basil leaves, for garnish (optional)

Instructions:

1. **Preheat Oven:** Preheat your oven to 375°F (190°C). Line a baking sheet with parchment paper.
2. **Make Meatballs:** In a bowl, combine the ground turkey, breadcrumbs, beaten egg, Parmesan cheese, oregano, salt, and pepper. Mix well. Form into small meatballs, about 1 inch in diameter, and place on the prepared baking sheet.
3. **Bake Meatballs:** Bake in the preheated oven for about 20-25 minutes, or until the meatballs are cooked through and lightly browned.
4. **Prepare Sauce:** While the meatballs are baking, heat the olive oil in a saucepan over medium heat. Add the onion and garlic, sautéing until soft and translucent, about 5 minutes. Add the tomato sauce, and simmer for 10-15 minutes. Season with salt and pepper to taste.
5. **Combine:** Add the baked meatballs to the sauce, gently stirring to coat. Simmer for an additional 5 minutes to allow the flavors to meld.
6. **Serve:** Divide the meatballs and sauce between plates or bowls. Garnish with fresh basil leaves if desired.

Nutritional Information: Calories: 360 | Carbs: 22g | Fat: 18g | Protein: 28g | Fibers: 3g

Tip: These turkey meatballs offer a high-protein, comforting meal, perfect for those in the recovery phase seeking gentle, nutritious options. The low-fiber tomato sauce is easy on the digestive system, while still providing the rich flavors of a traditional sauce. Adjust the seasoning and herbs in the sauce according to your preferences and dietary tolerances.

65. Soft-Cooked Vegetable Quiche without Crust

Prep Time: 10 minutes | **Cooking Time:** 30 minutes | **Servings:** 2

Ingredients:

- 4 large eggs
- 1 cup heavy cream
- 1/2 cup grated cheddar cheese
- 1/2 cup cooked vegetables (such as spinach, bell peppers, and zucchini, finely chopped and well-drained)
- Salt and pepper to taste
- A pinch of nutmeg (optional)

Instructions:

1. **Preheat Oven:** Preheat your oven to 375°F (190°C). Grease a 9-inch pie dish or a similar baking dish with a bit of butter or oil.

2. **Prepare Egg Mixture:** In a large bowl, whisk together the eggs, heavy cream, salt, pepper, and nutmeg until well combined.

3. **Add Vegetables and Cheese:** Stir in the cooked, drained vegetables and grated cheddar cheese into the egg mixture until evenly distributed.

4. **Bake:** Pour the mixture into the prepared pie dish. Place in the preheated oven and bake for 25-30 minutes, or until the quiche is set and the top is lightly golden.

5. **Cool and Serve:** Allow the quiche to cool for a few minutes before slicing and serving. This will help it set and make it easier to cut.

Nutritional Information: Calories: 580 | Carbs: 6g | Fat: 52g | Protein: 22g | Fibers: 1g

Tip: This crustless quiche is a wonderful low-fiber option that's rich in protein and adaptable to include your choice of soft-cooked vegetables. The absence of a crust makes it easier to digest, and it's a versatile dish that can be enjoyed at any meal. Feel free to adjust the types of vegetables and cheese based on your preferences and what's gentle on your stomach.

66. Poached Pear Salad with Walnut Dressing

Prep Time: 15 minutes | **Cooking Time:** 20 minutes | **Servings:** 2

Ingredients:

- 2 ripe pears, peeled, halved, and cored
- 2 cups water
- 1/4 cup white sugar
- 1 cinnamon stick
- **For the Salad:**
  - Mixed greens (optional, ensure they're tolerated, or use spinach for a softer option)
- **For the Walnut Dressing:**
  - 1/4 cup walnuts, finely chopped
  - 2 tablespoons olive oil
  - 1 tablespoon balsamic vinegar
  - 1 teaspoon honey
  - Salt and pepper to taste

Instructions:

1. **Poach Pears:** In a saucepan, combine water, sugar, and cinnamon stick. Bring to a simmer. Add pear halves and simmer gently for about 15-20 minutes, or until tender but still holding their shape. Remove pears from liquid and let cool. Slice thinly.

2. **Prepare Walnut Dressing:** In a small bowl, whisk together olive oil, balsamic vinegar, honey, and chopped walnuts. Season with salt and pepper to taste.

3. **Assemble Salad:** Arrange mixed greens or spinach on plates. Top with sliced poached pears.

4. **Serve:** Drizzle walnut dressing over the salad and pears before serving.

Nutritional Information: Calories: 300 | Carbs: 38g | Fat: 18g | Protein: 2g | Fibers: 5g

Tip: This elegant salad combines the sweet, soft texture of poached pears with a rich, nutty walnut dressing. It's a light and digestible option suitable for the recovery phase, offering a mix of textures and flavors without overwhelming your digestive system. Adjust the ingredients based on your dietary needs and preferences.

67. Mashed Root Vegetables with Grilled Chicken Breast

Prep Time: 15 minutes | **Cooking Time:** 30 minutes | **Servings:** 2

Ingredients:

- 2 chicken breasts
- 1 tablespoon olive oil
- Salt and pepper to taste
- 1 cup carrots, peeled and chopped
- 1 cup parsnips, peeled and chopped
- 1 cup turnips, peeled and chopped
- 2 tablespoons unsalted butter
- 1/4 cup milk or cream
- Fresh thyme or parsley, chopped for garnish (optional)

Instructions:

1. **Preheat Grill:** Preheat your grill or grill pan over medium-high heat. Brush the chicken breasts with olive oil and season with salt and pepper.

2. **Grill Chicken:** Grill the chicken breasts for about 6-7 minutes per side, or until fully cooked and an internal temperature of 165°F (74°C) is reached. Remove from the grill and let rest for a few minutes before slicing.

3. **Cook Root Vegetables:** While the chicken is grilling, place the chopped carrots, parsnips, and turnips in a large pot. Cover with water and bring to a boil. Reduce heat to medium and simmer for 20 minutes, or until the vegetables are very tender.

4. **Mash Vegetables:** Drain the cooked vegetables and return them to the pot. Add butter and milk (or cream), and mash the vegetables until smooth. Season with salt and pepper to taste.

5. **Serve:** Divide the mashed root vegetables between two plates. Top with sliced grilled chicken breast. Garnish with fresh thyme or parsley if desired.

Nutritional Information: Calories: 420 | Carbs: 34g | Fat: 18g | Protein: 35g | Fibers: 8g

Tip: This meal pairs the lean protein of grilled chicken with the sweet, earthy flavors of mashed root vegetables, making it a hearty yet easily digestible option for dinner. The root vegetables provide a comforting texture and can be a gentle way to include some fiber in your recovery diet. Adjust the creaminess of the mash with more or less milk or butter to suit your preference.

68. Creamy Risotto with Parmesan and Spinach

Prep Time: 5 minutes | **Cooking Time:** 25 minutes | **Servings:** 2

Ingredients:

- 1 cup Arborio rice
- 4 cups low-sodium chicken or vegetable broth, warmed
- 1 small onion, finely chopped
- 2 cloves garlic, minced
- 1 tablespoon olive oil
- 1/2 cup grated Parmesan cheese
- 1 cup fresh spinach leaves, roughly chopped
- Salt and pepper to taste
- 1 tablespoon unsalted butter

Instructions:

1. **Sauté Onion and Garlic:** In a large saucepan, heat the olive oil over medium heat. Add the onion and garlic, sautéing until soft and translucent, about 3-4 minutes.

2. **Cook Risotto:** Add the Arborio rice to the saucepan, stirring for about 1 minute to coat the rice with the oil. Begin adding the warm broth, one ladle at a time, stirring frequently. Wait until the liquid is almost fully absorbed before adding the next ladle. Continue this process until the rice is creamy and just tender, about 20 minutes.

3. **Add Spinach and Cheese:** Stir in the chopped spinach and grated Parmesan cheese until the spinach is wilted and the cheese is melted into the risotto. Season with salt and pepper to taste.

4. **Finish with Butter:** Remove from heat and stir in the butter until melted and incorporated into the risotto.

5. **Serve:** Divide the risotto between two bowls, garnishing with additional Parmesan cheese if desired.

Nutritional Information: Calories: 510 | Carbs: 70g | Fat: 18g | Protein: 18g | Fibers: 3g

Tip: This creamy risotto offers a comforting and nutritious meal, perfect for the recovery phase. The spinach provides a gentle way to incorporate greens into your diet, while the Parmesan adds a rich depth of flavor. For a softer texture, ensure the rice is thoroughly cooked and creamy.

69. Stewed Beef with Pumpkin Puree

Prep Time: 15 minutes | **Cooking Time:** 2 hours | **Servings:** 2

Ingredients:

- 1/2 pound beef stew meat, cut into cubes
- 2 tablespoons olive oil
- 1 small onion, finely chopped
- 2 cloves garlic, minced
- 2 cups beef broth
- 1 cup pumpkin puree (canned or homemade)
- 1/2 teaspoon dried thyme
- Salt and pepper to taste
- Fresh parsley, chopped for garnish (optional)

Instructions:

1. **Brown the Beef:** In a large pot or Dutch oven, heat 1 tablespoon of olive oil over medium-high heat. Add the beef cubes and cook until browned on all sides. Remove the beef and set aside.
2. **Sauté Onion and Garlic:** In the same pot, add the remaining olive oil. Add the chopped onion and garlic, cooking until softened, about 3-4 minutes.
3. **Combine Ingredients:** Return the beef to the pot. Add the beef broth, pumpkin puree, and dried thyme. Season with salt and pepper. Stir to combine all the ingredients.
4. **Simmer:** Bring the mixture to a simmer, then reduce the heat to low. Cover and let it cook for about 2 hours, or until the beef is tender and the stew has thickened.
5. **Serve:** Check the seasoning and adjust if necessary. Divide the stew between two bowls and garnish with chopped parsley if using.

Nutritional Information: Calories: 440 | Carbs: 15g | Fat: 25g | Protein: 35g | Fibers: 3g

Tip: This hearty stew combines tender beef with the sweetness of pumpkin for a comforting, nutritious meal suitable for the recovery phase. The slow cooking process ensures the beef is soft and easy to digest, while the pumpkin puree adds a creamy texture and a boost of vitamins.

70.   Broccoli and Cauliflower Cheese Bake

Prep Time: 15 minutes | **Cooking Time:** 25 minutes | **Servings:** 2

Ingredients:

- 1 cup broccoli florets, cut into small pieces
- 1 cup cauliflower florets, cut into small pieces
- 1 tablespoon olive oil
- Salt and pepper to taste
- 1 cup milk
- 2 tablespoons unsalted butter
- 2 tablespoons all-purpose flour
- 1 cup grated cheddar cheese
- 1/4 teaspoon ground nutmeg (optional)
- Bread crumbs for topping (optional, use gluten-free if necessary)

Instructions:

1. **Preheat Oven:** Preheat your oven to 375°F (190°C). Lightly grease a baking dish.
2. **Blanch Vegetables:** Bring a large pot of salted water to a boil. Add the broccoli and cauliflower florets and blanch for 2 minutes. Drain and set aside.
3. **Make Cheese Sauce:** In a saucepan, melt the butter over medium heat. Whisk in the flour to form a roux. Gradually add the milk, whisking constantly, until the mixture is smooth and thickened. Stir in the grated cheddar cheese until melted and smooth. Season with salt, pepper, and nutmeg if using.
4. **Combine:** In the prepared baking dish, combine the blanched broccoli and cauliflower. Pour the cheese sauce over the vegetables, ensuring they are well coated. If using, sprinkle bread crumbs on top for a crunchy finish.
5. **Bake:** Bake in the preheated oven for 20-25 minutes, or until the top is golden brown and bubbly.
6. **Serve:** Let the bake cool for a few minutes before serving to allow the sauce to set slightly.

Nutritional Information: Calories: 450 | Carbs: 22g | Fat: 34g | Protein: 20g | Fibers: 4g

Tip: This comforting bake combines the nutritional benefits of broccoli and cauliflower with the creamy, cheesy goodness of a homemade sauce. It's a warm, comforting dish suitable for those in the recovery phase who can tolerate dairy and are looking for a more indulgent way to consume vegetables. The blanching step ensures the vegetables are tender and easier to digest.

Chapter 5: Maintenance Phase: High-Fiber Recipes

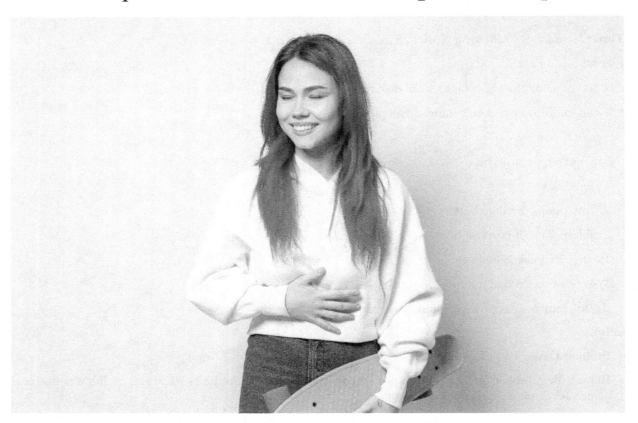

This chapter serves as your guide to thriving in the maintenance phase of diverticulitis, a crucial stage where the focus shifts from recovery to long-term management and prevention of future flare-ups. This chapter is filled with recipes that not only cater to the nutritional needs crucial for maintaining a healthy digestive system but also celebrate the joy of eating with a variety of flavors and textures that enrich your daily meals.

As you transition into this phase, the emphasis on a high-fiber diet becomes paramount. A diverse intake of fiber-rich foods is essential for supporting digestive health, regulating bowel movements, and preventing the recurrence of diverticulitis symptoms. However, it's also important to balance this with the understanding that every individual's tolerance to fiber varies, and adjustments may be necessary based on personal response.

- **Diverse Fiber Sources**: The recipes in this chapter highlight a wide array of fiber-rich ingredients, from fruits and vegetables to whole grains and legumes. Each recipe is designed to introduce these foods in delicious and digestible ways, ensuring you can meet your fiber goals without compromise.
- **Probiotic-Rich Foods**: Recognizing the role of gut microbiota in overall digestive health, this chapter includes meals that incorporate probiotic-rich foods, such as yogurt and kefir, which can help maintain a healthy balance of gut bacteria.
- **Balanced, Nutritious Meals**: Beyond fiber, these recipes ensure a balanced intake of proteins, healthy fats, and carbohydrates. This holistic approach supports not only your digestive system but your overall health, providing the energy and nutrients your body needs to thrive.
- **Mindful Meal Planning**: With an eye towards long-term maintenance, this chapter also touches on strategies for mindful meal planning. It includes tips for diversifying your diet, managing portion sizes, and incorporating new foods gradually to gauge their impact on your digestive system.

As you explore these recipes, remember that the journey with diverticulitis is deeply personal, and flexibility and patience are key to finding the dietary balance that works best for you.

Breakfast Recipes

71. Mixed Berry and Chia Seed Parfait

Prep Time: 10 minutes | **No Cooking Required** | **Servings:** 2

Ingredients:

- 1 cup Greek yogurt
- 2 tablespoons chia seeds
- 1 tablespoon honey, plus more for drizzling
- 1/2 cup mixed berries (such as strawberries, blueberries, and raspberries)
- 1/4 cup granola

Instructions:

1. **Prepare Chia Mixture:** In a small bowl, mix together the Greek yogurt, chia seeds, and 1 tablespoon of honey. Stir well until the honey is fully incorporated. Let the mixture sit for about 5 minutes to allow the chia seeds to swell.
2. **Assemble Parfait:** Spoon half of the chia-yogurt mixture into two glasses or parfait cups. Add a layer of mixed berries on top of the chia mixture in each glass. Sprinkle a layer of granola over the berries.
3. **Repeat Layers:** Repeat the layering with the remaining chia-yogurt mixture and berries. Optionally, you can add another layer of granola if you prefer more crunch.
4. **Serve:** Drizzle with a little more honey on top before serving, if desired.

Nutritional Information: Calories: 280 | Carbs: 36g | Fat: 10g | Protein: 15g | Fibers: 7g

Tip: This parfait combines the creaminess of Greek yogurt with the crunch of granola and the natural sweetness of berries, enhanced by the nutritional boost of chia seeds. It's a balanced, high-fiber breakfast that's both nutritious and delicious, perfect for starting your day in the maintenance phase of diverticulitis. You can customize this parfait with your favorite berries and granola to suit your taste preferences.

72. Whole Grain Toast with Avocado Spread

Prep Time: 5 minutes | **No Cooking Required** | **Servings:** 2

Ingredients:

- 2 slices whole grain bread
- 1 ripe avocado
- Salt and pepper to taste
- Red pepper flakes (optional)
- 1 teaspoon lemon juice
- 1 tablespoon pumpkin seeds (optional)

Instructions:

1. **Prepare Avocado Spread:** Cut the avocado in half and remove the pit. Scoop the flesh into a bowl and mash it with a fork until it reaches your desired consistency. Stir in the lemon juice, and season with salt, pepper, and red pepper flakes if using.

2. **Toast Bread:** Toast the whole grain bread slices to your liking.

3. **Assemble:** Spread the mashed avocado evenly over the toasted bread slices.

4. **Garnish:** Sprinkle pumpkin seeds over the avocado spread for added texture and a nutritional boost, if desired.

5. **Serve:** Enjoy immediately for the best taste and texture.

Nutritional Information: Calories: 320 | Carbs: 37g | Fat: 17g | Protein: 9g | Fibers: 10g

Tip: This simple yet satisfying breakfast option combines the heart-healthy fats of avocado with the fiber-rich benefits of whole grain bread. The lemon juice adds a fresh zing that complements the creamy avocado, while pumpkin seeds offer a crunchy texture and are a good source of minerals. This dish is perfect for maintaining a high-fiber diet in the maintenance phase of diverticulitis.

73. Oatmeal with Fresh Fruit and Almonds

Prep Time: 5 minutes | **Cooking Time:** 5 minutes | **Servings:** 2

Ingredients:

- 1 cup rolled oats

- 2 cups water or milk (for a creamier texture)

- Pinch of salt

- 1/2 cup mixed fresh fruit (such as blueberries, sliced strawberries, and banana slices)

- 2 tablespoons sliced almonds

- 1 tablespoon honey or maple syrup (optional)

- 1/2 teaspoon ground cinnamon (optional)

Instructions:

1. **Cook Oatmeal:** In a medium saucepan, bring the water or milk to a boil. Add a pinch of salt and the rolled oats. Reduce the heat to medium-low and simmer, stirring occasionally, until the oats are soft and have absorbed most of the liquid, about 5 minutes.

2. **Prepare Fruit and Almonds:** While the oatmeal is cooking, prepare your fresh fruit and measure out the sliced almonds.

3. **Serve:** Divide the cooked oatmeal into two bowls. Top each bowl with an equal amount of fresh fruit and sliced almonds. Drizzle with honey or maple syrup and sprinkle with cinnamon if using.

4. **Enjoy:** Serve warm for a comforting and nutritious start to your day.

Nutritional Information: Calories: 300 | Carbs: 45g | Fat: 9g | Protein: 10g | Fibers: 7g

Tip: This oatmeal recipe is a versatile and heart-healthy option for the maintenance phase, allowing you to incorporate a variety of fiber-rich fruits and nuts. The almonds add a crunchy texture and are a good source of healthy fats. Feel free to customize the toppings based on seasonal availability or personal preference to maintain a balanced and enjoyable high-fiber diet.

74. Spinach and Feta Whole Wheat Muffins

Prep Time: 15 minutes | **Cooking Time:** 20 minutes | **Servings:** 6 muffins

Ingredients:

- 1 cup whole wheat flour
- 1 teaspoon baking powder
- 1/2 teaspoon salt
- 2 large eggs
- 1/4 cup olive oil
- 1/2 cup milk
- 1 cup fresh spinach, finely chopped
- 1/2 cup feta cheese, crumbled
- 1/4 cup sun-dried tomatoes, chopped (optional)

Instructions:

1. **Preheat Oven and Prepare Muffin Tin:** Preheat your oven to 375°F (190°C). Line a muffin tin with paper liners or lightly grease the cups.
2. **Mix Dry Ingredients:** In a large bowl, whisk together the whole wheat flour, baking powder, and salt.
3. **Combine Wet Ingredients:** In another bowl, beat the eggs with the olive oil and milk until well combined.
4. **Add Wet to Dry:** Pour the wet ingredients into the dry ingredients, stirring just until combined. Be careful not to overmix.
5. **Fold in Extras:** Gently fold the chopped spinach, crumbled feta cheese, and sun-dried tomatoes (if using) into the batter.
6. **Fill Muffin Cups and Bake:** Divide the batter evenly among the prepared muffin cups, filling each about two-thirds full. Bake in the preheated oven for 20 minutes, or until a toothpick inserted into the center of a muffin comes out clean.
7. **Cool and Serve:** Allow the muffins to cool in the pan for a few minutes, then transfer them to a wire rack to cool completely. Serve warm or at room temperature.

Nutritional Information: Calories: 220 | Carbs: 20g | Fat: 13g | Protein: 7g | Fibers: 3g

Tip: These savory muffins offer a delightful combination of flavors and textures, with the whole wheat flour providing a hearty base, the spinach adding a fresh note, and the feta cheese giving a tangy kick. They're a great way to incorporate more whole grains and vegetables into your breakfast or as a snack during the maintenance phase of a high-fiber diet. Plus, they're portable and convenient for on-the-go eating.

75. Quinoa Breakfast Bowl with Berries

Prep Time: 5 minutes | **Cooking Time:** 15 minutes | **Servings:** 2

Ingredients:

- 1 cup quinoa, rinsed
- 2 cups water
- 1/2 cup mixed berries (such as blueberries, raspberries, and sliced strawberries)
- 2 tablespoons chopped nuts (such as almonds or walnuts)
- 1 tablespoon honey or maple syrup (optional)
- A pinch of cinnamon (optional)
- 2 tablespoons Greek yogurt (optional)

Instructions:

1. **Cook Quinoa:** In a medium saucepan, bring the 2 cups of water to a boil. Add the rinsed quinoa and a pinch of salt. Reduce the heat to low, cover, and simmer for about 15 minutes, or until all the water is absorbed and the quinoa is tender. Remove from heat and let it stand covered for 5 minutes. Fluff with a fork.
2. **Assemble the Bowl:** Divide the cooked quinoa into two bowls. Top each bowl with an equal amount of mixed berries and chopped nuts. Drizzle with honey or maple syrup and sprinkle with cinnamon if using.
3. **Add Greek Yogurt:** Add a dollop of Greek yogurt on top of each bowl for extra creaminess and a protein boost, if desired.
4. **Serve:** Enjoy this nutritious and flavorful quinoa breakfast bowl warm or at room temperature.

Nutritional Information: Calories: 310 | Carbs: 55g | Fat: 8g | Protein: 11g | Fibers: 6g

Tip: This quinoa breakfast bowl is a fiber-rich start to your day, packed with the nutritional benefits of quinoa and fresh berries. Quinoa is a complete protein, offering all nine essential amino acids, making this dish a powerful fuel for your morning. The addition of nuts adds healthy fats and extra texture, while Greek yogurt can provide a probiotic boost.

76. Whole Grain Pancakes with Maple Syrup

Prep Time: 10 minutes | **Cooking Time:** 15 minutes | **Servings:** 2

Ingredients:

- 1 cup whole grain flour (such as whole wheat or spelt flour)
- 1 tablespoon baking powder
- 1/4 teaspoon salt
- 1 cup milk (dairy or plant-based)
- 1 egg
- 2 tablespoons melted unsalted butter or coconut oil, plus more for cooking
- 1 tablespoon maple syrup, plus more for serving
- Fresh berries for topping (optional)

Instructions:

1. **Mix Dry Ingredients:** In a large bowl, whisk together the whole grain flour, baking powder, and salt.

2. **Combine Wet Ingredients:** In another bowl, beat the milk, egg, melted butter (or coconut oil), and maple syrup until well combined.

3. **Make Pancake Batter:** Pour the wet ingredients into the dry ingredients, stirring just until the mixture is combined and no large lumps remain. Be careful not to overmix.

4. **Cook Pancakes:** Heat a non-stick skillet or griddle over medium heat and brush with a little butter or oil. Pour 1/4 cup of batter for each pancake onto the hot skillet. Cook until bubbles form on the surface of the pancake, then flip and cook until golden brown on the other side, about 2-3 minutes per side.

5. **Serve:** Serve the pancakes warm, topped with additional maple syrup and fresh berries if desired.

Nutritional Information: Calories: 320 | Carbs: 48g | Fat: 10g | Protein: 10g | Fibers: 6g

Tip: These whole grain pancakes are a delicious way to enjoy a high-fiber breakfast that doesn't compromise on flavor or texture. The whole grains provide sustained energy and help support digestive health during the maintenance phase of diverticulitis. Serving with fresh berries not only adds a burst of flavor but also increases the fiber content and adds antioxidants to your meal.

77. Baked Sweet Potato and Black Bean Hash

Prep Time: 10 minutes | **Cooking Time:** 25 minutes | **Servings:** 2

Ingredients:

- 2 medium sweet potatoes, peeled and diced

- 1 tablespoon olive oil

- Salt and pepper to taste

- 1/2 cup black beans, rinsed and drained

- 1/2 red bell pepper, diced

- 1/2 onion, diced

- 1 teaspoon ground cumin

- 2 eggs (optional, for topping)

- Fresh cilantro, chopped for garnish (optional)

- Avocado slices for serving (optional)

Instructions:

1. **Preheat Oven and Roast Sweet Potatoes:** Preheat your oven to 400°F (200°C). Toss the diced sweet potatoes with olive oil, salt, and pepper on a baking sheet. Spread in a single layer and roast for about 20 minutes, or until tender and beginning to brown.

2. **Sauté Vegetables:** While the sweet potatoes are roasting, heat a skillet over medium heat. Add a little more olive oil, then sauté the onion and red bell pepper until soft, about 5 minutes. Stir in the black beans and ground cumin, cooking for an additional 2 minutes. Season with salt and pepper to taste.

3. **Combine Hash:** Add the roasted sweet potatoes to the skillet with the black bean mixture, gently mixing to combine.

4. **Cook Eggs (Optional):** In another skillet, fry the eggs to your liking. Season with salt and pepper.

5. **Serve:** Divide the sweet potato and black bean hash between plates. Top each with a fried egg, if using, and garnish with chopped cilantro and avocado slices.

Nutritional Information: Calories: 360 | Carbs: 55g | Fat: 10g | Protein: 12g | Fibers: 10g

Tip: This hearty and nutritious hash combines the natural sweetness of sweet potatoes with the fiber and protein of black beans, making it an excellent breakfast option for the maintenance phase of a high-fiber diet. The addition of a fried egg on top adds protein and richness, turning it into a complete meal. Adjust the level of spices to suit your taste and dietary tolerance.

78. Greek Yogurt Smoothie with Mixed Berries

Prep Time: 5 minutes | **Total Time:** 5 minutes | **Servings:** 2

Ingredients:

- 1 cup Greek yogurt, plain
- 1 cup mixed berries (strawberries, blueberries, raspberries), fresh or frozen
- 1 banana, sliced
- 1/2 cup almond milk, unsweetened
- 1 tablespoon honey or maple syrup (optional)
- 1 tablespoon chia seeds (optional)

Instructions:

1. **Blend Ingredients:** In a blender, combine the Greek yogurt, mixed berries, banana, almond milk, and honey or maple syrup if using. Blend until smooth. If the smoothie is too thick, you can add a little more almond milk to reach your desired consistency.

2. **Add Chia Seeds:** If using chia seeds, add them after blending and stir well. Let the smoothie sit for a few minutes to allow the chia seeds to swell and thicken the smoothie slightly.

3. **Serve:** Pour the smoothie into glasses and serve immediately. You can garnish with a few whole berries on top for a decorative touch.

Nutritional Information: Calories: 220 | Carbs: 36g | Fat: 4g | Protein: 12g | Fibers: 6g

Tip: This smoothie is a fantastic way to start your day with a boost of protein from Greek yogurt and a healthy dose of antioxidants from the mixed berries. The addition of chia seeds not only thickens the smoothie but also adds fiber and omega-3 fatty acids, making it a powerhouse of nutrition suitable for the maintenance phase of diverticulitis.

79. Vegetable and Goat Cheese Frittata

Prep Time: 10 minutes | **Cooking Time:** 20 minutes | **Servings:** 2

Ingredients:

- 4 large eggs
- 1/4 cup milk
- Salt and pepper to taste
- 2 tablespoons olive oil
- 1/2 cup cherry tomatoes, halved
- 1/2 cup spinach, roughly chopped
- 1/4 cup bell pepper, diced
- 1/4 cup goat cheese, crumbled
- Fresh herbs (such as basil or chives), for garnish

Instructions:

1. **Preheat the Oven:** Preheat your oven to 375°F (190°C).
2. **Whisk Eggs:** In a bowl, whisk together the eggs, milk, salt, and pepper until well combined.
3. **Sauté Vegetables:** In an ovenproof skillet, heat the olive oil over medium heat. Add the cherry tomatoes, spinach, and bell pepper. Sauté for about 3-4 minutes, or until the vegetables are just softened.
4. **Add Egg Mixture:** Pour the egg mixture over the sautéed vegetables in the skillet. Stir gently to ensure the vegetables are evenly distributed.
5. **Add Goat Cheese:** Sprinkle the crumbled goat cheese over the top of the egg mixture.
6. **Bake:** Transfer the skillet to the preheated oven. Bake for 12-15 minutes, or until the frittata is set and the top is lightly golden.
7. **Serve:** Let the frittata cool for a couple of minutes, then garnish with fresh herbs before slicing and serving.

Nutritional Information: Calories: 320 | Carbs: 8g | Fat: 24g | Protein: 20g | Fibers: 2g

Tip: This frittata combines the nutritional benefits of eggs with a variety of vegetables and the creamy tang of goat cheese, making it a flavorful and satisfying meal. It's a versatile dish that can be adapted to include any vegetables you have on hand, making it perfect for a high-fiber diet in the maintenance phase of diverticulitis.

80. Banana and Walnut Whole Wheat Bread

Prep Time: 15 minutes | **Cooking Time:** 55 minutes | **Servings:** 1 loaf

Ingredients:

- 1 3/4 cups whole wheat flour
- 1 teaspoon baking soda
- 1/2 teaspoon salt
- 1/3 cup unsalted butter, melted
- 1/2 cup honey or maple syrup
- 2 large eggs
- 1 cup mashed ripe bananas (about 2-3 bananas)
- 1/4 cup milk (dairy or plant-based)
- 1 teaspoon vanilla extract
- 1/2 cup walnuts, chopped (optional)

Instructions:

1. **Preheat Oven and Prepare Pan:** Preheat your oven to 325°F (165°C). Grease a 9x5 inch loaf pan or line it with parchment paper.
2. **Mix Dry Ingredients:** In a large bowl, whisk together the whole wheat flour, baking soda, and salt.
3. **Combine Wet Ingredients:** In another bowl, mix the melted butter and honey (or maple syrup). Add the eggs, one at a time, beating well after each addition. Stir in the mashed bananas, milk, and vanilla extract until well combined.
4. **Combine Wet and Dry Mixtures:** Add the wet ingredients to the dry ingredients, stirring just until combined and no dry spots remain. Gently fold in the chopped walnuts, if using.
5. **Bake:** Pour the batter into the prepared loaf pan. Bake in the preheated oven for 55-60 minutes, or until a toothpick inserted into the center comes out clean.
6. **Cool:** Let the bread cool in the pan for 10 minutes, then transfer it to a wire rack to cool completely.

Nutritional Information: Calories: 210 (per slice, based on 10 slices) | Carbs: 32g | Fat: 8g | Protein: 4g | Fibers: 4g

Tip: This banana and walnut whole wheat bread is a hearty, nutritious option for breakfast or a snack. The whole wheat flour and bananas provide a good source of dietary fiber, while the walnuts add healthy fats and a crunchy texture. Enjoy a slice with a cup of tea or coffee for a satisfying start to your day.

Snack Recipes

81. Crunchy Chickpea and Kale Chips

Prep Time: 10 minutes | **Cooking Time:** 20 minutes | **Servings:** 4

Ingredients:

- 1 can (15 oz) chickpeas, drained and rinsed
- 2 cups kale leaves, torn into bite-sized pieces
- 1 tablespoon olive oil
- 1/2 teaspoon salt
- 1/4 teaspoon garlic powder
- 1/4 teaspoon smoked paprika (optional)

Instructions:

1. **Preheat the Oven:** Preheat your oven to 400°F (200°C). Line a baking sheet with parchment paper.
2. **Prepare Chickpeas and Kale:** Pat the chickpeas dry with a paper towel. In a large bowl, toss the chickpeas and kale leaves with olive oil, ensuring they are evenly coated. Sprinkle with salt, garlic powder, and smoked paprika, if using.
3. **Bake:** Spread the chickpeas and kale leaves in a single layer on the prepared baking sheet. Bake for 15-20 minutes, or until the chickpeas are crispy and the kale chips are lightly browned and crisp.
4. **Cool and Serve:** Allow the chickpea and kale chips to cool slightly on the baking sheet for a few minutes before serving. This will help them crisp up even more.

Nutritional Information: Calories: 150 | Carbs: 20g | Fat: 6g | Protein: 7g | Fibers: 5g

Tip: This crunchy snack is perfect for the maintenance phase, offering a high-fiber, nutritious alternative to traditional chips. The combination of chickpeas and kale provides both a satisfying crunch and a boost of essential nutrients, making it a great snack to support digestive health.

82. Almond and Flaxseed Energy Balls

Prep Time: 15 minutes | **Chill Time:** 30 minutes | **Servings:** 12 balls

Ingredients:

- 1 cup almonds
- 1/4 cup flaxseeds
- 1/2 cup dates, pitted
- 2 tablespoons honey or maple syrup
- 1 teaspoon vanilla extract
- A pinch of salt

Instructions:

1. **Process Almonds and Flaxseeds:** In a food processor, blend the almonds and flaxseeds until they reach a coarse meal consistency.

2. **Add Remaining Ingredients:** Add the dates, honey or maple syrup, vanilla extract, and a pinch of salt to the food processor. Process until the mixture sticks together when pressed.

3. **Form Energy Balls:** Scoop out tablespoon-sized amounts of the mixture and roll them into balls using your hands. If the mixture is too sticky, wet your hands slightly before rolling.

4. **Chill:** Place the energy balls on a baking sheet lined with parchment paper. Refrigerate for at least 30 minutes to firm up.

5. **Serve:** Enjoy the energy balls as a quick and nutritious snack. Store any leftovers in an airtight container in the refrigerator.

Nutritional Information: Calories: 120 | Carbs: 10g | Fat: 8g | Protein: 3g | Fibers: 3g

Tip: These almond and flaxseed energy balls are a fantastic high-fiber snack for the maintenance phase, delivering a healthy blend of fats, protein, and fiber. They're perfect for an on-the-go energy boost or a post-workout snack.

83. Whole Grain Crackers with Spicy Hummus

Prep Time: 10 minutes | **Cooking Time:** 0 minutes | **Servings:** 4

Ingredients:

- 1 cup store-bought or homemade spicy hummus
- 20 whole grain crackers

Instructions:

1. **Prepare Hummus:** If you're making homemade hummus, blend chickpeas, tahini, lemon juice, garlic, and your choice of spices (such as cumin and chili powder) until smooth. For a spicy kick, add a diced jalapeño or a dash of cayenne pepper.

2. **Serve:** Spread the spicy hummus on whole grain crackers. Arrange on a platter for serving.

3. **Garnish (optional):** For extra flavor and color, garnish the hummus-topped crackers with a sprinkle of paprika, chopped parsley, or sliced olives.

Nutritional Information: Calories: 150 | Carbs: 20g | Fat: 7g | Protein: 5g | Fibers: 4g

Tip: This snack combines the satisfying crunch of whole grain crackers with the bold flavors of spicy hummus, making it an excellent high-fiber choice for the maintenance phase. It's perfect for midday snacking or as a healthy appetizer.

84. Fresh Veggie Sticks with Avocado Dip

Prep Time: 15 minutes | **Cooking Time:** 0 minutes | **Servings:** 4

Ingredients:

- 2 ripe avocados
- 1 tablespoon lime juice
- 1/4 teaspoon salt
- 1/4 teaspoon garlic powder

- 1/4 cup cilantro, finely chopped (optional)
- 1 carrot, peeled and cut into sticks
- 1 cucumber, cut into sticks
- 1 bell pepper, cut into sticks
- 1 celery stalk, cut into sticks

Instructions:

1. **Make the Avocado Dip:** In a medium bowl, mash the avocados with a fork. Stir in lime juice, salt, garlic powder, and cilantro (if using) until well combined and smooth.
2. **Prepare the Veggies:** Wash and cut the carrot, cucumber, bell pepper, and celery into stick shapes suitable for dipping.
3. **Serve:** Arrange the veggie sticks on a platter around the bowl of avocado dip. Enjoy dipping the fresh veggies into the creamy avocado mixture.

Nutritional Information: Calories: 200 | Carbs: 14g | Fat: 15g | Protein: 3g | Fibers: 7g

Tip: This refreshing snack is a powerhouse of nutrients and fibers, ideal for the maintenance phase of diverticulitis. The avocado dip provides healthy fats, while the assortment of veggie sticks offers a crunchy, hydrating way to enjoy a variety of vegetables. It's perfect for an afternoon pick-me-up or a healthy party platter.

85. Raspberry and Chia Seed Pudding

Prep Time: 10 minutes | **Chill Time:** 4 hours or overnight | **Servings:** 2

Ingredients:

- 1/4 cup chia seeds
- 1 cup almond milk (or any milk of your choice)
- 1 tablespoon maple syrup (adjust to taste)
- 1/2 teaspoon vanilla extract
- 1/2 cup fresh raspberries (plus extra for garnish)

Instructions:

1. **Mix Ingredients:** In a bowl, combine chia seeds, almond milk, maple syrup, and vanilla extract. Stir well to ensure the mixture is well combined and the chia seeds are fully submerged in the liquid.
2. **Add Raspberries:** Gently fold in the raspberries, being careful not to crush them completely.
3. **Chill:** Cover the bowl with a lid or plastic wrap and refrigerate for at least 4 hours, or overnight, until the pudding has thickened and the chia seeds have absorbed the liquid, creating a gel-like consistency.
4. **Serve:** Once set, stir the pudding, and divide it into serving bowls or glasses. Garnish with additional raspberries on top.
5. **Enjoy:** The pudding can be enjoyed immediately or stored in the refrigerator for up to 3 days.

Nutritional Information: Calories: 180 | Carbs: 24g | Fat: 8g | Protein: 5g | Fibers: 10g

Tip: This raspberry and chia seed pudding is a delightful, fiber-rich snack ideal for the maintenance phase of diverticulitis. Chia seeds provide a substantial fiber boost, while raspberries add natural sweetness and antioxidant benefits. It's a perfect make-ahead snack that's both nutritious and satisfying.

Lunch Recipes

86. Mediterranean Quinoa Salad with Chickpeas

Prep Time: 15 minutes | **Cooking Time:** 15 minutes | **Servings:** 2

Ingredients:

- 1 cup quinoa, rinsed
- 2 cups water
- 1 can (15 oz) chickpeas, rinsed and drained
- 1 cup cherry tomatoes, halved
- 1 cucumber, diced
- 1/2 red onion, finely chopped
- 1/4 cup kalamata olives, halved
- 1/4 cup feta cheese, crumbled
- **For the Dressing:**
    - 3 tablespoons olive oil
    - 2 tablespoons lemon juice
    - 1 garlic clove, minced
    - 1 teaspoon dried oregano
    - Salt and pepper to taste

Instructions:

1. **Cook Quinoa:** In a medium saucepan, bring the 2 cups of water to a boil. Add the quinoa and a pinch of salt. Reduce the heat to low, cover, and simmer for about 15 minutes, or until all the water is absorbed. Remove from heat, fluff with a fork, and let cool.
2. **Prepare Dressing:** In a small bowl, whisk together the olive oil, lemon juice, minced garlic, dried oregano, salt, and pepper until well combined.
3. **Combine Salad Ingredients:** In a large bowl, combine the cooled quinoa, chickpeas, cherry tomatoes, cucumber, red onion, kalamata olives, and feta cheese.
4. **Toss with Dressing:** Pour the dressing over the salad and toss to evenly coat all the ingredients.
5. **Serve:** The salad can be served immediately or chilled in the refrigerator for an hour to allow the flavors to meld.

Nutritional Information: Calories: 420 | Carbs: 55g | Fat: 18g | Protein: 14g | Fibers: 10g

Tip: This vibrant and nutritious Mediterranean quinoa salad is packed with flavors and textures. It's a perfect high-fiber lunch that combines the health benefits of quinoa and chickpeas with the fresh, crisp vegetables and the tangy feta cheese. Ideal for the maintenance phase, this salad offers a balanced meal that supports digestive health.

87. Grilled Chicken Caesar Wrap with Whole Wheat Tortilla

Prep Time: 20 minutes | **Cooking Time:** 10 minutes | **Servings:** 2

Ingredients:

- 2 whole wheat tortillas
- 2 chicken breasts, boneless and skinless
- Salt and pepper to taste
- 1 tablespoon olive oil
- 1/2 cup Caesar salad dressing, light or homemade
- 2 cups romaine lettuce, chopped
- 1/4 cup Parmesan cheese, shredded
- 1/4 cup whole grain croutons, crushed (optional)

Instructions:

1. **Prep Chicken:** Season chicken breasts with salt and pepper. Brush them with olive oil.
2. **Grill Chicken:** Preheat a grill or grill pan over medium-high heat. Grill the chicken for 5 minutes on each side, or until fully cooked through and juices run clear. Let it rest for a few minutes, then slice thinly.
3. **Warm Tortillas:** Warm the whole wheat tortillas in a dry skillet or in the microwave for a few seconds to make them more pliable.
4. **Assemble Wraps:** Spread Caesar salad dressing over each tortilla. Add a layer of chopped romaine lettuce, followed by sliced grilled chicken and shredded Parmesan cheese. Sprinkle crushed croutons over the top if using.
5. **Roll and Serve:** Roll up the tortillas tightly, tucking in the edges. Cut in half and serve immediately.

Nutritional Information: Calories: 550 | Carbs: 40g | Fat: 25g | Protein: 45g | Fibers: 6g

Tip: This wrap offers a healthier take on the classic Caesar salad by incorporating grilled chicken and whole wheat tortillas for added fiber and protein. It's a convenient and flavorful lunch option that balances creamy dressing with the crunch of lettuce and croutons. For a lighter version, look for a reduced-fat Caesar dressing or make your own with Greek yogurt.

88. Roasted Vegetable and Hummus Pita Pockets

Prep Time: 15 minutes | **Cooking Time:** 25 minutes | **Servings:** 2

Ingredients:

- 1 small zucchini, sliced
- 1 small yellow squash, sliced
- 1 red bell pepper, sliced
- 1 tablespoon olive oil
- Salt and pepper to taste
- 2 whole wheat pita breads
- 1/2 cup hummus
- Fresh spinach leaves (optional)

Instructions:

1. **Roast Vegetables:** Preheat your oven to 425°F (220°C). Toss the zucchini, yellow squash, and red bell pepper with olive oil, salt, and pepper on a baking sheet. Spread in a single layer and roast for about 20-25 minutes, or until vegetables are tender and lightly browned.
2. **Prepare Pita Pockets:** While the vegetables are roasting, cut the whole wheat pita breads in half to create pockets. If desired, you can lightly toast the pita halves to make them more pliable.
3. **Assemble Pita Pockets:** Spread a generous layer of hummus inside each pita half. Fill with the roasted vegetables, and add fresh spinach leaves if using.
4. **Serve:** Enjoy the pita pockets immediately while the vegetables are still warm, or allow them to cool to room temperature.

Nutritional Information: Calories: 330 | Carbs: 45g | Fat: 14g | Protein: 12g | Fibers: 8g

Tip: These pita pockets are a delicious and nutritious lunch option, combining the rich flavors of roasted vegetables with the creamy texture of hummus. Whole wheat pita provides additional fiber, making this meal both satisfying and supportive of a high-fiber diet. The hummus can also contribute to your intake of plant-based protein and healthy fats.

89. Kale and Quinoa Salad with Lemon Tahini Dressing

Prep Time: 15 minutes | **Cooking Time:** 15 minutes | **Servings:** 2

Ingredients:

- 1/2 cup quinoa, rinsed
- 1 cup water
- 2 cups kale, stems removed and leaves finely chopped
- 1/2 avocado, diced
- 1/4 cup cucumber, diced
- 1/4 cup cherry tomatoes, halved
- 2 tablespoons red onion, finely chopped

- 2 tablespoons almonds, sliced or chopped
- **For the Lemon Tahini Dressing:**
  - 2 tablespoons tahini
  - 1 tablespoon lemon juice
  - 1 clove garlic, minced
  - 2-4 tablespoons water, as needed to thin
  - Salt and pepper to taste

Instructions:

1. **Cook Quinoa:** In a medium saucepan, bring 1 cup of water to a boil. Add the quinoa and a pinch of salt, reduce the heat to low, cover, and simmer for about 15 minutes, or until the water is absorbed. Remove from heat, fluff with a fork, and let cool.

2. **Prepare Dressing:** In a small bowl, whisk together tahini, lemon juice, minced garlic, and enough water to reach your desired dressing consistency. Season with salt and pepper to taste.

3. **Assemble Salad:** In a large bowl, combine the cooled quinoa, chopped kale, diced avocado, cucumber, cherry tomatoes, red onion, and almonds. Toss with the lemon tahini dressing until everything is evenly coated.

4. **Serve:** Divide the salad between two plates or bowls and serve immediately.

Nutritional Information: Calories: 370 | Carbs: 45g | Fat: 18g | Protein: 12g | Fibers: 9g

Tip: This hearty salad is a powerhouse of nutrition, featuring a blend of high-fiber ingredients like kale and quinoa, healthy fats from avocado and tahini, and the crunch of almonds. The lemon tahini dressing adds a creamy, zesty finish that brings all the flavors together. It's a perfect, refreshing meal for the maintenance phase, offering both taste and health benefits.

90. Turkey and Avocado Club Sandwich on Multigrain Bread

Prep Time: 10 minutes | **No Cooking Required** | **Servings:** 2

Ingredients:

- 4 slices multigrain bread, lightly toasted
- 6 ounces sliced turkey breast
- 1 ripe avocado, mashed
- 2 lettuce leaves, washed and dried
- 4 slices tomato
- 2 tablespoons mayonnaise (or a healthier alternative like avocado mayo)
- Salt and pepper to taste
- 4 slices cooked bacon (optional for extra crunch and flavor)

Instructions:

1. **Prepare Ingredients:** Lightly toast the multigrain bread slices. Mash the avocado in a small bowl and season with a little salt and pepper.

2. **Assemble Sandwiches:** Spread mayonnaise on one side of each bread slice. On two of the slices, layer half the mashed avocado, followed by turkey slices, lettuce, tomato slices, and bacon if using. Season each layer lightly with salt and pepper as desired.

3. **Complete and Serve:** Top each sandwich with another slice of bread, mayonnaise side down. Carefully cut each sandwich in half or into quarters for easier eating.

4. **Enjoy:** Serve immediately, offering a balance of lean protein, healthy fats, and high-fiber from the multigrain bread and vegetables.

Nutritional Information: Calories: 450 | Carbs: 38g | Fat: 20g | Protein: 32g | Fibers: 8g

Tip: This modern take on the classic club sandwich incorporates healthy, fiber-rich ingredients without sacrificing flavor. The multigrain bread and avocado add important nutrients and fibers, supporting your dietary goals in the maintenance phase of diverticulitis. The combination of textures, from creamy avocado to crisp lettuce and optional bacon, makes this sandwich a satisfying meal.

91. Black Bean and Corn Taco Salad with Whole Grain Chips

Prep Time: 15 minutes | **No Cooking Required** | **Servings:** 2

Ingredients:

- 1 can (15 oz) black beans, rinsed and drained
- 1 cup corn kernels, fresh or thawed from frozen
- 1/2 cup cherry tomatoes, quartered
- 1/4 cup red onion, finely chopped
- 1 avocado, diced
- 1/2 cup cilantro, chopped
- Juice of 1 lime
- Salt and pepper to taste
- 1 teaspoon ground cumin
- 2 cups romaine lettuce, chopped
- Whole grain tortilla chips for serving
- Optional: Shredded cheese, sour cream, or Greek yogurt for topping

Instructions:

1. **Mix Salad Ingredients:** In a large bowl, combine the black beans, corn, cherry tomatoes, red onion, diced avocado, and chopped cilantro.

2. **Dress the Salad:** Add the lime juice, salt, pepper, and ground cumin to the salad. Toss everything together until well mixed.

3. **Prepare Lettuce Base:** Place a bed of chopped romaine lettuce on each plate.

4. **Assemble Salad:** Spoon the black bean and corn mixture over the lettuce.

5. **Add Crunch:** Break whole grain tortilla chips into large pieces and sprinkle them over the top of the salad.

6. **Add Toppings:** If desired, top the salad with shredded cheese, a dollop of sour cream, or Greek yogurt.

7. **Serve:** Enjoy this refreshing and fiber-rich taco salad immediately for the best combination of flavors and textures.

Nutritional Information: Calories: 400 | Carbs: 55g | Fat: 15g | Protein: 15g | Fibers: 15g

Tip: This taco salad is a flavorful, nutritious meal that combines the heartiness of black beans with the freshness of vegetables and the crunch of whole grain chips. It's a versatile recipe that can be easily adjusted to include your favorite taco toppings, making it perfect for a high-fiber lunch that supports digestive health in the maintenance phase of diverticulitis.

92. Whole Wheat Pasta Salad with Cherry Tomatoes and Feta

Prep Time: 10 minutes | **Cooking Time:** 10 minutes | **Servings:** 2

Ingredients:

- 8 ounces whole wheat pasta (such as fusilli or penne)
- 1 cup cherry tomatoes, halved
- 1/2 cup cucumber, diced
- 1/4 cup red onion, finely chopped
- 1/2 cup feta cheese, crumbled
- 1/4 cup black olives, sliced (optional)
- **For the Dressing:**
  - 3 tablespoons olive oil
  - 2 tablespoons balsamic vinegar
  - 1 teaspoon Dijon mustard
  - Salt and pepper to taste
  - Fresh basil leaves, chopped, for garnish

Instructions:

1. **Cook Pasta:** Cook the whole wheat pasta according to package instructions until al dente. Drain and rinse under cold water to cool. Transfer to a large mixing bowl.
2. **Prepare Dressing:** In a small bowl, whisk together the olive oil, balsamic vinegar, Dijon mustard, salt, and pepper until well combined.
3. **Combine Ingredients:** To the bowl with the pasta, add the halved cherry tomatoes, diced cucumber, finely chopped red onion, crumbled feta cheese, and sliced black olives if using.
4. **Toss with Dressing:** Pour the dressing over the pasta salad and toss to evenly coat all the ingredients.
5. **Serve:** Garnish the pasta salad with chopped fresh basil before serving. Can be enjoyed immediately or chilled in the refrigerator for 1 hour to allow flavors to meld.

Nutritional Information: Calories: 480 | Carbs: 68g | Fat: 18g | Protein: 16g | Fibers: 10g

Tip: This refreshing pasta salad is a delightful blend of textures and Mediterranean flavors, made healthier with whole wheat pasta for an added fiber boost. It's a versatile dish that can be served as a light lunch or a side, perfect for the maintenance phase of a high-fiber diet. Feel free to add more vegetables or a protein like grilled chicken to customize it to your taste.

93. Asian-inspired Tofu and Vegetable Stir Fry

Prep Time: 15 minutes | **Cooking Time:** 10 minutes | **Servings:** 2

Ingredients:

- 1 block (14 oz) firm tofu, pressed and cubed
- 2 tablespoons sesame oil
- 1 cup broccoli florets
- 1/2 red bell pepper, sliced
- 1/2 cup snap peas, trimmed
- 1 carrot, julienned
- 2 green onions, chopped
- 2 cloves garlic, minced
- 1 inch piece ginger, grated
- **For the Sauce:**
    - 3 tablespoons soy sauce (low sodium)
    - 1 tablespoon rice vinegar
    - 1 tablespoon honey or maple syrup
    - 1 teaspoon cornstarch (dissolved in 2 tablespoons water)
- Sesame seeds for garnish

Instructions:

1. **Prepare Tofu:** In a non-stick skillet or wok, heat 1 tablespoon sesame oil over medium-high heat. Add the tofu cubes and fry until golden on all sides. Remove tofu from the skillet and set aside.
2. **Stir Fry Vegetables:** In the same skillet, add the remaining sesame oil. Sauté the broccoli, red bell pepper, snap peas, carrot, green onions, garlic, and ginger for about 5 minutes, or until the vegetables are just tender but still crisp.
3. **Make Sauce:** In a small bowl, whisk together the soy sauce, rice vinegar, honey or maple syrup, and dissolved cornstarch.
4. **Combine Tofu and Vegetables with Sauce:** Return the tofu to the skillet with the vegetables. Pour the sauce over the tofu and vegetables, stirring to combine. Cook for another 2-3 minutes, until the sauce has thickened and everything is heated through.
5. **Serve:** Divide the stir fry between two plates or bowls. Garnish with sesame seeds before serving.

Nutritional Information: Calories: 360 | Carbs: 24g | Fat: 20g | Protein: 22g | Fibers: 4g

Tip: This vibrant, Asian-inspired stir fry combines protein-rich tofu with a medley of colorful vegetables, all coated in a savory and slightly sweet sauce. It's a balanced, high-fiber meal that's perfect for the maintenance phase, offering a delicious way to enjoy a variety of vegetables in your diet. Adjust the level of sweetness or add a kick with some chili flakes or hot sauce to suit your taste.

94. Lentil Soup with Spinach and Carrots

Prep Time: 10 minutes | **Cooking Time:** 30 minutes | **Servings:** 2

Ingredients:

- 1 cup red lentils, rinsed
- 4 cups vegetable broth
- 1 medium carrot, diced
- 1/2 onion, chopped
- 2 cloves garlic, minced
- 1 teaspoon ground cumin
- 1/2 teaspoon ground turmeric (optional)
- Salt and pepper to taste
- 2 cups fresh spinach, roughly chopped
- 1 tablespoon olive oil
- Lemon wedges for serving

Instructions:

1. **Sauté Vegetables:** In a large pot, heat the olive oil over medium heat. Add the onion and garlic, and sauté until the onion is translucent, about 3-4 minutes. Add the diced carrot and cook for an additional 2 minutes.
2. **Cook Lentils:** Stir in the red lentils, vegetable broth, cumin, and turmeric (if using). Season with salt and pepper. Bring to a boil, then reduce the heat to low, cover, and simmer for about 20 minutes, or until the lentils are soft and the soup has thickened.
3. **Add Spinach:** Add the chopped spinach to the pot and cook for another 2-3 minutes, or until the spinach has wilted.
4. **Serve:** Ladle the soup into bowls. Serve with lemon wedges on the side for a fresh, bright flavor boost.

Nutritional Information: Calories: 340 | Carbs: 54g | Fat: 8g | Protein: 20g | Fibers: 14g

Tip: This hearty and nutritious lentil soup is enriched with the goodness of spinach and carrots, offering a high-fiber, plant-based protein meal that's perfect for the maintenance phase. The spices add depth and warmth, making it a comforting dish for any day. Adjust the seasoning to your taste, and don't hesitate to experiment with other vegetables you enjoy.

95. Grilled Salmon Salad with Mixed Greens and Vinaigrette

Prep Time: 15 minutes | **Cooking Time:** 10 minutes | **Servings:** 2

Ingredients:

- 2 salmon fillets (about 6 ounces each)
- Salt and pepper to taste
- 1 tablespoon olive oil
- 4 cups mixed greens (such as arugula, spinach, and romaine)
- 1/2 cup cherry tomatoes, halved
- 1/4 red onion, thinly sliced
- 1/4 cucumber, sliced
- **For the Vinaigrette:**
  - 3 tablespoons extra virgin olive oil
  - 1 tablespoon balsamic vinegar
  - 1 teaspoon Dijon mustard
  - Salt and pepper to taste

Instructions:

1. **Prep Salmon:** Season the salmon fillets with salt and pepper. Brush them lightly with olive oil.
2. **Grill Salmon:** Preheat a grill or grill pan over medium-high heat. Grill the salmon for about 5 minutes on each side, or until cooked through and easily flaked with a fork. Let it cool slightly, then flake into large pieces.
3. **Make Vinaigrette:** In a small bowl, whisk together the extra virgin olive oil, balsamic vinegar, Dijon mustard, salt, and pepper until well combined.
4. **Assemble Salad:** In a large bowl, toss the mixed greens, cherry tomatoes, red onion, and cucumber with the vinaigrette. Divide the salad between two plates.
5. **Top with Salmon:** Place the flaked salmon on top of the salads.
6. **Serve:** Enjoy the salad immediately, offering a perfect balance of lean protein, fresh vegetables, and a tangy dressing.

Nutritional Information: Calories: 420 | Carbs: 8g | Fat: 28g | Protein: 34g | Fibers: 2g

Tip: This grilled salmon salad is a delightful blend of flavors and textures, providing a nutrient-dense meal that supports a high-fiber diet in the maintenance phase of diverticulitis. The omega-3 fatty acids in the salmon contribute to heart health, while the mixed greens offer a variety of vitamins and minerals. Adjust the components of the vinaigrette to match your personal taste preferences.

Dinner Recipes

96. Stuffed Bell Peppers with Brown Rice and Turkey

Prep Time: 20 minutes | **Cooking Time:** 40 minutes | **Servings:** 2

Ingredients:

- 2 large bell peppers, halved and seeded
- 1/2 cup brown rice, cooked
- 1/2 pound ground turkey
- 1 tablespoon olive oil
- 1/2 onion, diced
- 2 cloves garlic, minced
- 1 cup spinach, chopped
- 1/4 cup tomato sauce
- 1/4 cup low-sodium chicken or vegetable broth
- 1/2 teaspoon cumin
- Salt and pepper to taste
- 1/4 cup shredded mozzarella cheese (optional)
- Fresh parsley, chopped for garnish

Instructions:

1. **Preheat Oven:** Preheat your oven to 375°F (190°C).
2. **Prepare Peppers:** Arrange the bell pepper halves in a baking dish, cut-side up.
3. **Cook Turkey:** In a skillet over medium heat, heat the olive oil. Add the ground turkey, season with salt and pepper, and cook until browned. Set aside.
4. **Sauté Vegetables:** In the same skillet, add the onion and garlic, cooking until softened. Add the chopped spinach and cook until wilted. Mix in the cooked brown rice, tomato sauce, cooked turkey, cumin, salt, and pepper.
5. **Stuff Peppers:** Spoon the turkey and rice mixture evenly into the bell pepper halves. Pour the broth into the bottom of the baking dish around the peppers.
6. **Bake:** Cover with foil and bake for about 30 minutes. Uncover, sprinkle with mozzarella cheese if using, and bake for another 10 minutes, or until the peppers are tender and the cheese is melted and lightly browned.
7. **Serve:** Garnish with fresh parsley before serving.

Nutritional Information: Calories: 450 | Carbs: 40g | Fat: 18g | Protein: 35g | Fibers: 6g

Tip: These stuffed bell peppers are a hearty, nutritious meal that combines lean protein, whole grains, and vegetables in one dish. The brown rice provides a fiber boost, while the turkey and vegetables ensure you're getting a variety of nutrients. This meal is satisfying and balanced, perfect for the maintenance phase of diverticulitis.

97. Eggplant and Chickpea Curry with Quinoa

Prep Time: 15 minutes | **Cooking Time:** 30 minutes | **Servings:** 2

Ingredients:

- 1 cup quinoa, rinsed
- 2 cups water or vegetable broth
- 1 tablespoon olive oil
- 1 small eggplant, diced into cubes
- 1 can (15 oz) chickpeas, drained and rinsed
- 1 onion, finely chopped
- 2 cloves garlic, minced
- 1 tablespoon curry powder
- 1 teaspoon ground turmeric
- 1 can (14 oz) diced tomatoes
- 1 can (14 oz) coconut milk
- Salt and pepper to taste
- Fresh cilantro, for garnish
- Lemon wedges, for serving

Instructions:

1. **Cook Quinoa:** In a medium saucepan, bring the water or vegetable broth to a boil. Add the rinsed quinoa and a pinch of salt. Reduce the heat to low, cover, and simmer for 15-20 minutes, or until all the liquid is absorbed. Fluff with a fork and set aside.

2. **Sauté Vegetables:** In a large skillet or saucepan, heat the olive oil over medium heat. Add the onion and garlic, and sauté until softened, about 3-4 minutes. Add the eggplant cubes and cook, stirring occasionally, until they start to soften, about 5 minutes.

3. **Add Spices and Chickpeas:** Stir in the curry powder and turmeric until the vegetables are well coated. Add the chickpeas, diced tomatoes with their juice, and coconut milk. Season with salt and pepper.

4. **Simmer:** Bring the mixture to a simmer, then reduce the heat and continue to cook, uncovered, for about 20 minutes, or until the eggplant is tender and the sauce has thickened.

5. **Serve:** Spoon the eggplant and chickpea curry over the cooked quinoa. Garnish with fresh cilantro and serve with lemon wedges on the side.

Nutritional Information: Calories: 620 | Carbs: 80g | Fat: 25g | Protein: 18g | Fibers: 15g

Tip: This flavorful curry combines nutritious ingredients like eggplant and chickpeas with the complete protein source of quinoa, making it an excellent high-fiber dinner option. The rich, aromatic spices not only add depth to the dish but also offer various health benefits. Adjust the level of curry powder to suit your taste preferences and heat tolerance.

98. Roasted Butternut Squash and Lentil Salad

Prep Time: 15 minutes | **Cooking Time:** 30 minutes | **Servings:** 2

Ingredients:

- 1 cup butternut squash, peeled and cubed
- 1 tablespoon olive oil
- Salt and pepper to taste
- 1/2 cup green or brown lentils, rinsed
- 2 cups vegetable broth or water
- 1/4 red onion, thinly sliced
- 2 cups mixed salad greens
- **For the Dressing:**
    - 2 tablespoons extra virgin olive oil
    - 1 tablespoon apple cider vinegar
    - 1 teaspoon Dijon mustard
    - 1 teaspoon honey or maple syrup
    - Salt and pepper to taste

Instructions:

1. **Roast Butternut Squash:** Preheat your oven to 425°F (220°C). Toss the butternut squash cubes with 1 tablespoon of olive oil, salt, and pepper on a baking sheet. Spread in a single layer and roast for about 25-30 minutes, or until tender and caramelized, stirring halfway through.

2. **Cook Lentils:** While the squash is roasting, combine the lentils and vegetable broth in a medium saucepan. Bring to a boil, then reduce heat and simmer, covered, for 20-25 minutes, or until lentils are tender but still hold their shape. Drain any excess liquid.

3. **Prepare Dressing:** In a small bowl, whisk together the extra virgin olive oil, apple cider vinegar, Dijon mustard, honey or maple syrup, salt, and pepper to create the dressing.

4. **Assemble Salad:** In a large bowl, combine the roasted butternut squash, cooked lentils, red onion, and mixed salad greens. Drizzle with the dressing and toss gently to combine.

5. **Serve:** Divide the salad between two plates or bowls and serve immediately, or let it sit for a few minutes to allow the flavors to meld together.

Nutritional Information: Calories: 400 | Carbs: 58g | Fat: 14g | Protein: 16g | Fibers: 18g

Tip: This hearty salad offers a wonderful mix of textures and flavors, with the earthiness of lentils and the sweetness of roasted butternut squash. It's a nutrient-dense meal that provides plenty of fiber and protein, making it an excellent choice for the maintenance phase of a high-fiber diet. The salad can be served warm or at room temperature, making it versatile for any season.

99. Baked Trout with Walnut and Herb Crust

Prep Time: 10 minutes | **Cooking Time:** 15 minutes | **Servings:** 2

Ingredients:

- 2 trout fillets (about 6 ounces each)
- Salt and pepper to taste
- 1/2 cup walnuts, finely chopped
- 2 tablespoons fresh parsley, finely chopped
- 1 tablespoon fresh dill, finely chopped
- 1 garlic clove, minced
- 2 tablespoons olive oil
- Lemon wedges for serving

Instructions:

1. **Preheat Oven:** Preheat your oven to 400°F (200°C). Line a baking sheet with parchment paper.
2. **Season Trout:** Season the trout fillets with salt and pepper on both sides and place them on the prepared baking sheet.
3. **Prepare Walnut Herb Crust:** In a small bowl, combine the finely chopped walnuts, parsley, dill, minced garlic, and 1 tablespoon of olive oil. Mix until the mixture is cohesive.
4. **Apply Crust to Trout:** Press the walnut herb mixture onto the top of each trout fillet, covering the surface evenly.
5. **Bake:** Drizzle the remaining olive oil over the crusted fillets. Bake in the preheated oven for about 12-15 minutes, or until the trout is cooked through and the crust is golden.
6. **Serve:** Transfer the baked trout to plates and serve immediately with lemon wedges on the side.

Nutritional Information: Calories: 390 | Carbs: 2g | Fat: 28g | Protein: 34g | Fibers: 1g

Tip: This baked trout recipe offers a delicious way to enjoy fish with a crunchy, nutty topping that adds both flavor and healthy fats. The herbs provide a fresh aroma and taste, enhancing the natural flavors of the trout. It's a simple yet elegant dish suitable for a high-fiber diet, offering a good balance of protein and omega-3 fatty acids. Serve with a side of roasted vegetables or a fresh salad for a complete meal.

100. Vegetarian Black Bean Enchiladas

Prep Time: 20 minutes | **Cooking Time:** 25 minutes | **Servings:** 2

Ingredients:

- 4 whole wheat tortillas
- 1 can (15 oz) black beans, rinsed and drained
- 1 cup corn kernels, fresh or frozen and thawed
- 1/2 cup red bell pepper, diced
- 1/2 onion, diced
- 1 teaspoon ground cumin
- 1/2 teaspoon chili powder
- Salt and pepper to taste
- 1 cup enchilada sauce
- 1/2 cup shredded cheddar or Mexican blend cheese
- Fresh cilantro, chopped for garnish
- Greek yogurt or sour cream, for serving (optional)

Instructions:

1. **Preheat Oven:** Preheat your oven to 375°F (190°C). Lightly grease a baking dish.
2. **Prepare Filling:** In a bowl, combine the black beans, corn, red bell pepper, onion, cumin, chili powder, salt, and pepper. Mix well.
3. **Assemble Enchiladas:** Lay out the whole wheat tortillas on a flat surface. Divide the bean and vegetable mixture evenly among the tortillas, placing the filling in a line down the center of each tortilla. Roll up the tortillas tightly and place seam-side down in the prepared baking dish.
4. **Add Sauce and Cheese:** Pour the enchilada sauce evenly over the rolled tortillas, making sure they are completely covered. Sprinkle the shredded cheese over the top.
5. **Bake:** Bake in the preheated oven for 25 minutes, or until the enchiladas are heated through and the cheese is melted and bubbly.
6. **Garnish and Serve:** Garnish the enchiladas with chopped cilantro. Serve hot, with Greek yogurt or sour cream on the side if desired.

Nutritional Information: Calories: 450 | Carbs: 65g | Fat: 14g | Protein: 20g | Fibers: 12g

Tip: These vegetarian enchiladas are a hearty, satisfying meal packed with fiber and protein from the black beans and vegetables. The whole wheat tortillas add an extra fiber boost, making this dish a great addition to a high-fiber diet. Customize the filling with any vegetables you like, or add some heat with diced jalapeños.

101.   Garlic Ginger Stir-Fried Vegetables with Tempeh

Prep Time: 15 minutes | **Cooking Time:** 10 minutes | **Servings:** 2

Ingredients:

- 8 ounces tempeh, cut into 1/2-inch cubes
- 2 tablespoons soy sauce (low sodium)
- 1 tablespoon sesame oil
- 1 tablespoon olive oil
- 2 cloves garlic, minced
- 1 inch piece of ginger, grated
- 1 red bell pepper, sliced
- 1 carrot, julienned
- 1 cup broccoli florets
- 1/2 cup snap peas
- 2 green onions, sliced
- Sesame seeds for garnish

Instructions:

1. **Marinate Tempeh:** In a bowl, toss the tempeh cubes with soy sauce. Let marinate for at least 10 minutes.
2. **Stir-Fry Tempeh:** Heat the sesame oil in a large skillet or wok over medium-high heat. Add the marinated tempeh and stir-fry until golden brown on all sides, about 5 minutes. Remove tempeh from the skillet and set aside.
3. **Stir-Fry Vegetables:** In the same skillet, heat the olive oil over medium-high heat. Add the garlic and ginger, sautéing for 30 seconds until fragrant. Add the red bell pepper, carrot, broccoli, and snap peas. Stir-fry for about 5 minutes, or until the vegetables are tender but still crisp.
4. **Combine:** Return the tempeh to the skillet with the vegetables. Add the green onions and toss everything together, heating through.
5. **Serve:** Divide the stir-fried vegetables and tempeh between two plates. Garnish with sesame seeds before serving.

Nutritional Information: Calories: 380 | Carbs: 26g | Fat: 22g | Protein: 24g | Fibers: 8g

Tip: This vibrant stir-fry combines nutrient-dense tempeh with a medley of colorful vegetables, all flavored with aromatic garlic and ginger. It's a high-fiber, high-protein dish that's perfect for the maintenance phase of a high-fiber diet. The tempeh not only adds a satisfying texture but also boosts the meal's protein content, making this dish both filling and nutritious. Adjust the variety of vegetables based on seasonality and preference to keep this meal exciting and new.

102.   Spaghetti Squash with Chunky Tomato Sauce and Olives

Prep Time: 10 minutes | **Cooking Time:** 40 minutes | **Servings:** 2

Ingredients:

- 1 medium spaghetti squash
- 1 tablespoon olive oil
- Salt and pepper to taste
- 2 cups chunky tomato sauce (homemade or high-quality store-bought)
- 1/2 cup black olives, sliced
- 1/4 cup fresh basil, chopped
- Grated Parmesan cheese (optional)

Instructions:

1. **Preheat Oven:** Preheat your oven to 400°F (200°C). Line a baking sheet with parchment paper.
2. **Prepare Spaghetti Squash:** Cut the spaghetti squash in half lengthwise and scoop out the seeds. Brush the inside of each half with olive oil and season with salt and pepper. Place squash halves cut-side down on the prepared baking sheet.
3. **Roast Squash:** Roast in the preheated oven for about 30-40 minutes, or until the flesh is tender and easily shreds with a fork.
4. **Prepare Tomato Sauce:** While the squash is roasting, warm the tomato sauce in a saucepan over medium heat. Stir in the sliced olives and simmer until heated through.
5. **Shred Squash:** Once the squash is cooked, let it cool for a few minutes, then use a fork to scrape the flesh into spaghetti-like strands.
6. **Serve:** Divide the spaghetti squash strands between plates. Top with the warm chunky tomato sauce and olives. Garnish with fresh basil and grated Parmesan cheese if desired.

Nutritional Information: Calories: 280 | Carbs: 40g | Fat: 12g | Protein: 6g | Fibers: 9g

Tip: This dish offers a low-carb, high-fiber alternative to traditional pasta dishes, utilizing spaghetti squash as a nutrient-dense base. The chunky tomato sauce and olives provide a robust flavor profile, while fresh basil adds a burst of freshness. This meal is both satisfying and aligned with the goals of a high-fiber diet in the maintenance phase of diverticulitis, promoting digestive health without sacrificing taste.

103.   Moroccan-Spiced Chicken with Couscous and Vegetables

Prep Time: 20 minutes | **Cooking Time:** 30 minutes | **Servings:** 2

Ingredients:

- 2 chicken breasts, boneless and skinless
- 1 tablespoon Moroccan spice blend (ras el hanout or a mix of cumin, coriander, cinnamon, and paprika)
- Salt and pepper to taste
- 1 tablespoon olive oil
- 1 cup whole wheat couscous

- 2 cups vegetable broth or water
- 1 medium carrot, diced
- 1 zucchini, diced
- 1/2 red bell pepper, diced
- 1/4 cup raisins
- 1/4 cup almonds, toasted and chopped
- Fresh cilantro, for garnish
- Lemon wedges, for serving

Instructions:

1. **Season Chicken:** Rub the chicken breasts with the Moroccan spice blend, salt, and pepper.

2. **Cook Chicken:** In a skillet over medium heat, heat the olive oil. Add the seasoned chicken and cook for about 5-7 minutes on each side, or until fully cooked through and golden brown. Remove from the skillet and let rest before slicing.

3. **Prepare Couscous:** In a saucepan, bring the vegetable broth to a boil. Stir in the couscous, cover, and remove from heat. Let stand for 5 minutes, then fluff with a fork.

4. **Sauté Vegetables:** In the same skillet used for chicken, add a bit more olive oil if necessary. Sauté the carrot, zucchini, and red bell pepper until tender. Stir in the raisins and heat through.

5. **Combine:** Mix the sautéed vegetables and toasted almonds with the couscous.

6. **Serve:** Divide the vegetable couscous mixture between plates. Top with sliced chicken breast. Garnish with fresh cilantro and serve with lemon wedges on the side.

Nutritional Information: Calories: 520 | Carbs: 65g | Fat: 14g | Protein: 38g | Fibers: 9g

Tip: This dish brings the flavors of Morocco to your table with a nutritious combination of spiced chicken, whole wheat couscous, and a medley of vegetables. It's a balanced meal that provides a good mix of protein, fiber, and essential vitamins. The raisins add a touch of sweetness that complements the spices, making it a delightful high-fiber dinner option.

104.   Zucchini Noodles with Avocado Pesto and Cherry Tomatoes

Prep Time: 15 minutes | **No Cooking Required** | **Servings:** 2

Ingredients:

- 2 large zucchinis
- 1 ripe avocado
- 1/2 cup fresh basil leaves
- 2 tablespoons pine nuts, plus more for garnish
- 1 garlic clove
- 2 tablespoons lemon juice
- 1/4 cup olive oil
- Salt and pepper to taste
- 1 cup cherry tomatoes, halved
- Grated Parmesan cheese, for serving (optional)

Instructions:

1. **Make Zucchini Noodles:** Use a spiralizer to turn the zucchinis into noodles. Place the noodles in a large bowl.
2. **Prepare Avocado Pesto:** In a food processor, blend the avocado, basil leaves, pine nuts, garlic, and lemon juice until smooth. Gradually add the olive oil while continuing to blend. Season with salt and pepper to taste.
3. **Combine:** Pour the avocado pesto over the zucchini noodles. Toss gently to ensure the noodles are evenly coated.
4. **Add Tomatoes:** Add the halved cherry tomatoes to the zucchini noodles and toss lightly.
5. **Serve:** Divide the zucchini noodle mixture between two plates. Garnish with additional pine nuts and grated Parmesan cheese if desired.

Nutritional Information: Calories: 380 | Carbs: 20g | Fat: 32g | Protein: 6g | Fibers: 8g

Tip: This vibrant and refreshing dish offers a light yet satisfying meal, perfect for a high-fiber dinner. The creamy avocado pesto provides healthy fats, while the zucchini noodles are a fantastic low-carb, high-fiber alternative to traditional pasta. This dish is a great way to enjoy the flavors of summer any time of the year.

105. Portobello Mushroom Steaks with Barley Pilaf

Prep Time: 15 minutes | **Cooking Time:** 30 minutes | **Servings:** 2

Ingredients:

- 4 large Portobello mushrooms, stems removed
- 2 tablespoons olive oil
- 2 tablespoons balsamic vinegar
- 1 teaspoon garlic powder
- Salt and pepper to taste
- **For the Barley Pilaf:**
  - 1 cup barley, rinsed
  - 2 1/2 cups vegetable broth
  - 1 tablespoon olive oil
  - 1 small onion, diced
  - 1 carrot, diced
  - 1/4 cup dried cranberries or raisins
  - 1/4 cup chopped walnuts or almonds (optional)
  - Fresh parsley, chopped for garnish

Instructions:

1. **Marinate Mushrooms:** In a small bowl, whisk together olive oil, balsamic vinegar, garlic powder, salt, and pepper. Brush the mixture over both sides of the Portobello mushrooms. Let them marinate for at least 15 minutes.
2. **Cook Barley:** In a saucepan, bring the vegetable broth to a boil. Add the barley, reduce heat to low, cover, and simmer for about 25-30 minutes, or until the barley is tender and the liquid is absorbed.
3. **Sauté Vegetables:** While the barley is cooking, heat 1 tablespoon of olive oil in a skillet over medium heat. Sauté the onion and carrot until softened, about 5 minutes. Stir this mixture into the cooked barley along with the dried cranberries and nuts if using.
4. **Grill Mushrooms:** Preheat a grill or grill pan over medium-high heat. Grill the marinated mushrooms for about 5 minutes on each side, or until tender and grill marks appear.
5. **Serve:** Spoon a generous amount of barley pilaf onto each plate. Top with grilled Portobello mushrooms. Garnish with fresh parsley before serving.

Nutritional Information: Calories: 520 | Carbs: 75g | Fat: 20g | Protein: 12g | Fibers: 15g

Tip: This hearty and satisfying meal pairs the meaty texture of Portobello mushrooms with the nuttiness of barley pilaf, creating a delicious and nutritious plant-based dinner option. The mushrooms serve as a low-calorie, high-fiber steak alternative, while the barley pilaf adds a comforting and fulfilling side. This dish is a great way to enjoy a variety of textures and flavors while maintaining a high-fiber diet.

Part III: Specialized Dietary Considerations and Meal Planning

Chapter 6:   Creating Your Diverticulitis Diet Plan

Navigating through the complexities of diverticulitis is much more than a journey from diagnosis to recovery; it is about embarking on a lifelong path of dietary mindfulness and adaptation that promotes your digestive health and overall well-being. This chapter is dedicated to guiding you through the creation of a personalized diverticulitis diet plan. It's about understanding that while certain foods may provide comfort and nourishment to some, they might trigger discomfort for others. Thus, we aim to arm you with the knowledge and tools necessary to tailor a diet plan that aligns perfectly with your unique dietary needs and lifestyle, ensuring that managing your condition becomes a seamless part of your daily routine.

Understanding Your Body

The first step in mastering your diverticulitis diet is to become deeply attuned to your body's signals. The way our bodies react to different foods can be incredibly personal, thus making it essential to identify which foods act as triggers and which bring comfort and relief. By meticulously keeping a food diary, you can chart your body's reactions to various foods, understanding patterns and pinpointing specific triggers. This diary becomes your most trusted guide, helping you navigate your diet with precision, avoiding flare-ups, and maintaining digestive harmony.

Personalizing Your Diet Plan

With the insights gleaned from your food diary in hand, you're now equipped to construct a diet plan that not only meets the nutritional guidelines outlined in previous chapters but also caters to your individual food tolerances and preferences. This chapter walks you through the process of balancing your intake of macronutrients and micronutrients to support not just your digestive health but your overall vitality. We delve into how to modify your diet based on the phase of diverticulitis you are experiencing, offering practical advice on selecting foods that will nourish and sustain you whether you're in the midst of a flare-up, on the road to recovery, or looking to maintain your health long-term.

Incorporating Variety and Nutrition

A key to successfully managing diverticulitis over the long haul is ensuring your diet remains varied and nutritionally dense, thereby avoiding monotony and ensuring your meals are both satisfying and healthful. We explore strategies for introducing a broad spectrum of foods into your diet, emphasizing the importance of variety in keeping your meals interesting and nutritionally balanced. From creative meal planning to the art of recipe modification, this section is filled with tips and tricks to enhance the diversity of your diet, ensuring it remains rich in the fiber and nutrients essential for managing diverticulitis.

Supplementation and Diverticulitis

While a diverse, high-fiber diet is the cornerstone of managing diverticulitis, there are instances where dietary supplements may be necessary to fill nutritional gaps, especially during flare-ups or due to dietary restrictions. Here, we discuss when and how fiber supplements, probiotics, and multivitamins might be incorporated into your diet plan. It's important to approach supplementation with caution, and we stress the importance of consulting with healthcare professionals to ensure that any supplements you consider are appropriate and beneficial for your specific situation.

Lifestyle Considerations

Your diet is just one piece of the puzzle when it comes to managing diverticulitis and promoting overall health. This section highlights how lifestyle factors, including stress levels, physical activity, and sleep patterns, play critical roles in digestive health. We offer advice on developing habits that complement your dietary efforts, such as engaging in regular exercise, practicing stress-reduction techniques, and ensuring adequate hydration and sleep. By adopting a holistic approach to health, you can enhance your body's ability to manage diverticulitis and improve your quality of life.

Eating Out and Social Events

Maintaining a diverticulitis-friendly diet doesn't mean isolating yourself from social gatherings or dining out. This section provides you with strategies for navigating restaurants and social events, ensuring you can enjoy these experiences without compromising your dietary goals. From learning how to make high-fiber choices at restaurants to communicating your dietary needs with hosts and staff, we equip you with the tools needed to stay on track, no matter the setting.

Adjusting and Evolving Your Diet Plan

As your journey with diverticulitis continues, so too will your dietary needs and preferences evolve. This chapter concludes with guidance on regularly reviewing and adjusting your diet plan to accommodate changes in your condition, lifestyle, and nutritional requirements. Emphasizing the importance of an open dialogue with healthcare providers, we encourage you to view your diet plan as a dynamic, evolving framework that can be adapted to support your health and well-being throughout your life.

Creating and adhering to a personalized diverticulitis diet plan is an empowering step towards managing your condition and enhancing your overall health. With patience, experimentation, and a willingness to learn, you can develop a dietary strategy that not only minimizes symptoms and flare.

Nourish & Flourish: 7-Day Diverticulitis Diet Plans

Embarking on a journey with diverticulitis requires not just understanding your condition, but also learning how to nourish your body in a way that supports healing and long-term wellness. The following 7-day meal plans are designed for each phase of diverticulitis management—acute, recovery, and maintenance—to offer you a structured approach to eating during these times.

Important Notes: Please remember, these meal plans serve as a guideline and starting point. The duration of each phase can vary significantly from person to person, and transitioning between phases should always be done under the guidance of a healthcare professional. Listen to your body and adjust these plans according to your specific needs, preferences, and any dietary advice given by your doctor or dietitian. Our goal is to provide you with the tools and inspiration to create a diet plan that not only addresses the challenges of diverticulitis but also enriches your overall health.

Please note also that the proposed meal plans, including snacks, are designed for medium-calorie diets. Should your dietary needs require more controlled calorie intake, feel free to adjust by omitting snacks as needed. Moreover, should any of the recipes not suit your taste preferences, or if you have allergies or intolerances to certain ingredients, they can be conveniently substituted with others from the same dietary phase section, ensuring your meal plan remains aligned with your health goals and personal needs.

Acute Phase 7-day Meal Plan

Day	Breakfast	Mid-Morning Snack	Lunch	Afternoon Snack	Dinner
1	Gentle Ginger Tea	Soothing Clear Broth Cubes	Clear Chicken Broth	Cooling Peppermint Tea Gelatin	Broth-Based Vegetable Soup
2	Soothing Rice Porridge	Gentle Apple and Cinnamon Compote	Tender Chicken Broth Soup	Simple Honey-Drizzled Poached Pears	Mashed Carrot Puree
3	Herbal Infusion Blend	Hydrating Herbal Ice Pops	Soft-Cooked Acorn Squash	Soothing Clear Broth Cubes	Pureed Pumpkin Soup
4	Basic Apple Gelatin	Cooling Peppermint Tea Gelatin	Clear Beef Broth	Gentle Apple and Cinnamon Compote	Steamed White Fish Fillet
5	Plain Rice Water	Simple Honey-Drizzled Poached Pears	Silky Potato Soup	Soothing Clear Broth Cubes	Butternut Squash Puree
6	Low-Fiber Cream of Wheat	Gentle Apple and Cinnamon Compote	Simple Poached Chicken Breast	Hydrating Herbal Ice Pops	Clear Tomato Broth
7	Simple Poached Pear	Cooling Peppermint Tea Gelatin	Low-Fiber Baked Apple	Simple Honey-Drizzled Poached Pears	Smooth Carrot and Ginger Soup

This 7-day meal plan for the acute phase of diverticulitis provides a variety of liquid and very low-fiber options to ease symptoms, offering different recipes for each part of the day to keep the diet as interesting as possible while adhering to dietary restrictions. Each recipe selected is designed to be gentle on the digestive system, helping to manage acute symptoms effectively.

Recovery Phase 7-day Meal Plan

Day	Breakfast	Mid-Morning Snack	Lunch	Afternoon Snack	Dinner
1	Creamy Oatmeal with Mashed Banana	Mild Avocado Mash on Toasted White Bread	Quinoa Salad with Roasted Vegetables	Baked Banana with a Dash of Cinnamon	Grilled Tilapia with Lemon Herb Dressing
2	Scrambled Eggs with Avocado	Low-Fiber Berry and Yogurt Parfait	Baked Sweet Potato with Cottage Cheese	Creamy Low-Fiber Pumpkin Smoothie	Roasted Carrot and Ginger Soup
3	Baked Pears with Honey	Soft-Cooked Apple and Pear Sauce	Pureed Butternut Squash Soup	Mild Avocado Mash on Toasted White Bread	Baked Cod with Soft Herbed Polenta
4	Cottage Cheese with Soft Peaches	Baked Banana with a Dash of Cinnamon	Soft-Cooked Chicken and Rice Bowl	Low-Fiber Berry and Yogurt Parfait	Soft-Cooked Vegetable Quiche without Crust
5	Rice Porridge with Maple Syrup	Creamy Low-Fiber Pumpkin Smoothie	Steamed Salmon with Mashed Cauliflower	Soft-Cooked Apple and Pear Sauce	Poached Pear Salad with Walnut Dressing
6	Smooth Peanut Butter on Toasted White Bread	Mild Avocado Mash on Toasted White Bread	Turkey and Avocado Wrap with Soft Tortilla	Baked Banana with a Dash of Cinnamon	Mashed Root Vegetables with Grilled Chicken Breast
7	Soft-Boiled Eggs with Saltine Crackers	Low-Fiber Berry and Yogurt Parfait	Low-Fiber Vegetable Stir-Fry with Tofu	Creamy Low-Fiber Pumpkin Smoothie	Creamy Risotto with Parmesan and Spinach

This 7-day meal plan for the recovery phase provides a balanced approach to reintroducing more solid foods into the diet, with a focus on low to moderate fiber options to support healing and ease the transition from the acute phase. Each day offers a variety of meals to ensure nutritional needs are met while catering to a recovering digestive system.

Maintenance Phase 7-day Meal Plan

Day	Breakfast	Mid-Morning Snack	Lunch	Afternoon Snack	Dinner
1	Mixed Berry and Chia Seed Parfait	Crunchy Chickpea and Kale Chips	Mediterranean Quinoa Salad with Chickpeas	Almond and Flaxseed Energy Balls	Eggplant and Chickpea Curry with Quinoa
2	Oatmeal with Fresh Fruit and Almonds	Whole Grain Crackers with Spicy Hummus	Grilled Chicken Caesar Wrap with Whole Wheat Tortilla	Fresh Veggie Sticks with Avocado Dip	Baked Trout with Walnut and Herb Crust
3	Whole Grain Toast with Avocado Spread	Almond and Flaxseed Energy Balls	Roasted Vegetable and Hummus Pita Pockets	Crunchy Chickpea and Kale Chips	Vegetarian Black Bean Enchiladas
4	Quinoa Breakfast Bowl with Berries	Fresh Veggie Sticks with Avocado Dip	Kale and Quinoa Salad with Lemon Tahini Dressing	Whole Grain Crackers with Spicy Hummus	Garlic Ginger Stir-Fried Vegetables with Tempeh
5	Whole Grain Pancakes with Maple Syrup	Crunchy Chickpea and Kale Chips	Turkey and Avocado Club Sandwich on Multigrain Bread	Almond and Flaxseed Energy Balls	Spaghetti Squash with Chunky Tomato Sauce and Olives
6	Spinach and Feta Whole Wheat Muffins	Fresh Veggie Sticks with Avocado Dip	Black Bean and Corn Taco Salad with Whole Grain Chips	Raspberry and Chia Seed Pudding	Moroccan-Spiced Chicken with Couscous and Vegetables
7	Baked Sweet Potato and Black Bean Hash	Whole Grain Crackers with Spicy Hummus	Whole Wheat Pasta Salad with Cherry Tomatoes and Feta	Crunchy Chickpea and Kale Chips	Zucchini Noodles with Avocado Pesto and Cherry Tomatoes

This 7-day meal plan for the maintenance phase is rich in high-fiber foods, aimed at sustaining digestive health and preventing the recurrence of diverticulitis. It incorporates a wide variety of flavors and textures to ensure meals remain enjoyable and nutritionally balanced, supporting a healthy lifestyle.

Chapter 7:   Recipes That Adapt With You

Transitioning through the phases of diverticulitis demands not only an understanding of your dietary needs but also a collection of recipes that can evolve with your journey. This chapter is dedicated to offering you adaptable recipes that cater to the acute, recovery, and maintenance phases, ensuring that your meals can be modified to suit your current condition without sacrificing taste or nutritional value.

Adaptable Foundation Recipes: The Heart of Flexibility

At the heart of this chapter are the adaptable foundation recipes, designed for versatility and ease of modification. These foundational dishes serve as a canvas, allowing for the addition or subtraction of ingredients based on your dietary phase and tolerance.

- **Versatile Vegetable Soup**: Starting with a gentle, aromatic vegetable broth, this soup can be transformed by blending for a smooth consistency during the acute phase or by adding fiber-rich vegetables and grains as you transition into recovery and maintenance. Key to this approach is the understanding of how cooking methods affect digestibility and nutrient availability.

Tailoring Textures and Flavors

An essential aspect of making meals adaptable is the skillful modification of textures and flavors to meet your body's needs without compromising enjoyment.

- **Texture Transformations**: For those in the acute or recovery phases, textures need to be softer and easier to digest. Techniques such as pureeing or simmering foods longer can make them more suitable. As your digestive system heals, you can reintroduce more varied textures, which are not only enjoyable but also beneficial for stimulating digestive function.

- **Flavor Adjustments**: Flavor is paramount, regardless of the dietary phase. Using herbs, spices, and cooking techniques like roasting or sautéing can enhance flavors without adding strain to the digestive system. During the acute phase, flavors should be mild and soothing, while more robust and diverse flavors can be reintroduced as your diet expands.

Phase-Specific Recipe Adaptations: Navigating the Journey

This section provides a roadmap for adjusting recipes through each phase of diverticulitis, ensuring that you have options that are both healing and satisfying.

- **From Liquids to Solids**: Detailed guidelines on how to transition from a liquid-based diet to incorporating solids offer a practical approach to gradually reintroducing a broader range of foods. Suggestions for smooth transitions, such as moving from broths to smooth soups and then to soups with soft-cooked ingredients, help manage the dietary shifts effectively.

Personalizing Your Plate: The Ultimate Goal

Empowering you to personalize your meals according to your current health status, preferences, and nutritional needs is the ultimate goal of this chapter.

- **Empowerment through Education**: Equipping you with the knowledge to understand how different foods and their preparation methods affect your digestive system allows for informed decisions about meal choices. This empowerment is crucial for long-term management and enjoyment of your diet.

- **Creative Culinary Freedom**: Encouraging creativity in the kitchen is vital for maintaining interest and satisfaction with your diet. Experimenting with flavors, textures, and ingredients within the guidelines of your current dietary phase can transform meal preparation from a chore into an enjoyable and rewarding activity.

This chapter aims to make your dietary management journey less daunting and more empowering. By providing recipes that adapt with you, we hope to inspire confidence in the kitchen, allowing you to enjoy delicious, healthful meals tailored to your body's needs at every step of your diverticulitis journey.

Part IV: Living Well With Diverticulitis

Chapter 8: Beyond Diet: Lifestyle Changes for Diverticulitis Management

Introduction: Holistic Health for Holistic Healing

Managing diverticulitis extends far beyond dietary adjustments. While food plays a crucial role in mitigating symptoms and preventing flare-ups, a holistic approach incorporating broader lifestyle changes can significantly enhance your quality of life and contribute to long-term health. This chapter explores key lifestyle factors that, when addressed, can synergistically support your journey with diverticulitis.

Stress Management: Soothing the Mind to Soothe the Gut

The link between stress and digestive health is well-documented. Stress can exacerbate digestive symptoms, triggering flare-ups and complicating recovery. Incorporating stress-reduction techniques into your daily routine can have profound effects on your diverticulitis management.

- **Mindfulness and Meditation**: Simple, daily practices can help reduce stress levels and promote a sense of calm, directly impacting gut health.

- **Physical Activity**: Engaging in regular, gentle exercise not only reduces stress but also supports digestive function and overall health.

Physical Activity: Keeping the Body Moving

Regular exercise plays a pivotal role in managing diverticulitis by enhancing bowel function, reducing pressure within the colon, and supporting weight management. Tailoring your exercise regimen to your condition's current stage is crucial.

- **During Flare-Ups**: Focus on gentle movements and stretching exercises that keep the body active without straining the digestive system.

- **Recovery and Maintenance Phases**: Gradually incorporate more vigorous activities such as walking, swimming, or cycling, always listening to your body's cues.

Sleep and Rest: Foundations of Healing

Adequate sleep and rest are fundamental components of managing any health condition, including diverticulitis. Quality sleep supports immune function, aids in the healing process, and can help regulate stress hormones.

- **Establishing a Sleep Routine**: Consistency in your sleep schedule can significantly improve sleep quality.

- **Creating a Restful Environment**: Minimize light and noise in your sleeping area, and consider practices like reading or deep breathing to ease the transition to sleep.

Hydration: The Essence of Digestive Health

While hydration is a dietary consideration, its importance merits separate emphasis. Adequate fluid intake is crucial for softening stools and promoting easy passage through the colon, reducing the risk of diverticula becoming inflamed.

- **Water is Key**: Aim for at least 8 glasses of water daily, more if you're active or in hot climates.

- **Limiting Caffeine and Alcohol**: These can contribute to dehydration and should be consumed in moderation, especially during flare-ups.

Community and Support: Navigating Together

Diverticulitis management can feel isolating, but finding a community of others who understand your experience can provide invaluable support and encouragement.

- **Support Groups**: Whether online or in-person, support groups offer a space to share experiences, tips, and encouragement.

- **Family and Friends**: Educating your close circle about your condition can help them provide the support you need, whether it's adapting meal plans or understanding your need for rest.

A Lifestyle Aligned

Adopting a comprehensive approach to managing diverticulitis, one that encompasses diet and broader lifestyle changes, offers the best path to maintaining health and preventing flare-ups. Each aspect of your lifestyle, from stress management to physical activity and sleep, plays a role in supporting your digestive health. This chapter provides the foundation for building a lifestyle that aligns with your needs and promotes long-term wellness.

Chapter 9: Navigating Challenges: Dining Out and Social Events

Introduction: Embracing Social Life with Confidence
Living with diverticulitis shouldn't mean missing out on the joys of dining out and attending social events. This chapter provides practical advice and strategies to enjoy social occasions while adhering to your dietary needs, ensuring that you can participate fully in life's celebrations without compromising your health.

Preparing for Dining Out
Eating at restaurants can be one of the biggest challenges for those managing diverticulitis due to the uncertainty about food ingredients and preparation methods.

- **Restaurant Research**: Look up menus online ahead of time and identify restaurants that offer diverticulitis-friendly options. Don't hesitate to call and ask about menu items or request special accommodations.

- **Communicating Your Needs**: Learn how to clearly and confidently communicate your dietary restrictions to servers and chefs. A simple explanation of your needs can go a long way in ensuring a safe and enjoyable dining experience.

Managing Social Gatherings
Social gatherings, from family dinners to holiday parties, are an integral part of life but can pose dietary challenges.

- **Host Awareness**: If you're attending a gathering, inform your host about your dietary needs well in advance. Offer to bring a dish that you know is safe for you to eat and share with others.

- **Strategic Eating**: Eat a small, safe meal before attending events to curb hunger and reduce the temptation to eat potentially problematic foods.

Alcohol and Beverages
Alcohol and certain beverages can trigger diverticulitis symptoms or interfere with your digestive health.

- **Safe Sipping**: Opt for water or other non-irritating drinks. If you choose to drink alcohol, do so in moderation, and be aware of how different types of alcohol affect you.

Navigating Buffets and Potlucks
Buffets and potlucks offer a variety of food choices, but they can also be a minefield for those with dietary restrictions.

- **Visual Inspection**: Survey the entire buffet or potluck table before making your selections. Choose simple dishes with identifiable ingredients that align with your dietary phase.

- **Portion Control**: Take small portions to sample how your body reacts to different foods, especially if you're trying something new.

Building Resilience
Encountering setbacks or accidentally consuming something that triggers symptoms is possible. Developing strategies to handle these situations with grace and resilience is key.

- **Immediate Response**: If you suspect you've eaten something problematic, revert to your safe, symptom-management diet as soon as possible.

- **Reflection and Recovery**: Reflect on the experience to identify what might have gone wrong and how you can prevent it in the future. Consider keeping a food diary to track your reactions to different foods and situations.

Thriving Socially with Diverticulitis

This chapter has armed you with strategies and insights to navigate dining out and social events confidently. Remember, living with diverticulitis doesn't have to limit your social life. With preparation, communication, and self-awareness, you can enjoy a vibrant social life while managing your condition effectively.

Conclusion

Empowering Your Journey with Knowledge and Flavor

As we close the pages of "Diverticulitis Cookbook for Beginners: Embrace Nutritious, Easy-to-Make Recipes to Heal Your Gut, Enhance Wellness, and Bring Delight to Every Mealtime," it's essential to reflect on the journey we've embarked upon together. This guide was more than a collection of recipes; it was a beacon of hope, a source of empowerment, and a testament to the resilience of the human spirit in the face of dietary challenges posed by diverticulitis.

Navigating through the stages of diverticulitis requires patience, understanding, and a willingness to adapt. From the acute phase of managing symptoms with a liquid diet to the recovery phase's careful reintroduction of fiber, and finally, to the long-term maintenance of a balanced, high-fiber diet, this cookbook has provided you with the tools to tailor your dietary approach to meet your body's needs at every step.

But beyond the recipes and dietary guidelines, this book aimed to underscore the importance of a holistic approach to health. Stress management, physical activity, adequate rest, and social engagement are all integral components of a comprehensive strategy for managing diverticulitis. These lifestyle factors work in concert with your diet to support your digestive health and overall well-being.

Remember, the path to managing diverticulitis is highly personal. What works for one individual may not work for another. The key is to listen to your body, communicate openly with your healthcare providers, and not be afraid to make adjustments to your diet and lifestyle as needed. Empowerment comes from knowledge—understanding your condition, knowing how different foods and activities affect you, and making informed choices that enhance your quality of life.

As you move forward, let this cookbook be a constant companion in your journey. Revisit the recipes, tips, and guidance as often as needed. Allow yourself the freedom to experiment in the kitchen, finding joy and satisfaction in meals that nourish both your body and soul.

Thank you for allowing us to be a part of your journey toward health and wellness. May the knowledge you've gained empower you to embrace each day with confidence, knowing that you have the tools to manage your diverticulitis and live a full, vibrant life.

Remember, every meal is an opportunity to nurture not just your body, but also your spirit. Here's to a future filled with health, happiness, and delicious food.

Appendices

Appendix A: Food Diary Template: To track symptoms and identify trigger foods

Maintaining a food diary is a powerful tool for managing diverticulitis. It can help you and your healthcare provider identify foods that trigger symptoms, understand the impact of diet on your condition, and make informed adjustments to your eating habits. This template is designed to make tracking your meals, symptoms, and well-being as straightforward as possible.

Daily Food Diary Template

Date: _____

Meal Times: Breakfast | Lunch | Dinner | Snacks

Foods Consumed: List all foods and beverages consumed at each meal, including portion sizes and ingredients in mixed dishes.

Symptoms Experienced: Note any symptoms experienced after meals, such as abdominal pain, bloating, or changes in bowel habits. Rate the severity of symptoms on a scale of 1 to 10.

Physical Activity: Document any physical activity or exercise, including the type and duration.

Stress Levels: Rate your stress levels on a scale of 1 to 10 and note any significant stressors.

Sleep Quality: Record how many hours of sleep you got and rate the quality of your sleep on a scale of 1 to 10.

Overall Well-being: Provide a general note on how you felt throughout the day, including energy levels and mood.

Additional Notes: Use this space for any other observations that might be relevant, such as eating out, attending social events, trying new foods, or starting new medications.

Tips for Keeping a Food Diary

- **Be Consistent:** Try to fill in your food diary every day to capture a complete picture of your diet and symptoms.

- **Be Detailed:** Include as much detail as possible about the foods you eat, such as cooking methods and ingredients in prepared meals.

- **Look for Patterns:** Over time, review your diary to identify patterns between what you eat and the symptoms you experience.

- **Share with Your Healthcare Provider:** Bring your food diary to appointments to discuss your findings and adjust your management plan as needed.

Your food diary is a personal tool that can evolve with your journey managing diverticulitis. It's not just about tracking what you eat; it's about understanding the relationship between your diet, your body, and your well-being. Use this template as a stepping stone toward taking control of your diverticulitis and living a healthier, happier life.

Appendix B: Quick Reference Guide for Stage-Specific Foods

Understanding what to eat during each phase of diverticulitis can be challenging. This quick reference guide is designed to simplify the process, providing you with a go-to list of foods that are suitable for the acute phase, recovery phase, and maintenance phase of diverticulitis. Use this guide to help make informed dietary choices and navigate your meals with confidence.

Acute Phase: Soothing and Gentle

During a diverticulitis flare-up, your diet should be as gentle on your digestive system as possible. Focus on clear liquids and gradually transition to very low-fiber foods as your symptoms begin to subside.

- **Clear Liquids**: Water, clear broths, herbal teas, and electrolyte solutions.

- **Very Low-Fiber Foods** (as symptoms improve): Applesauce, boiled potatoes without skin, white rice.

Recovery Phase: Gradual Reintroduction

As you recover, you can start to reintroduce more fiber into your diet, but it's important to do so gradually and monitor how your body responds.

- **Low-Fiber Foods**: Canned or cooked fruits without skins or seeds, cooked tender vegetables, eggs, white bread.

- **Transition Foods**: Oatmeal, bananas, soft-cooked carrots, and beets; these foods provide a gentle reintroduction to fiber.

Maintenance Phase: Diverse and Balanced

In the maintenance phase, aim for a diverse, high-fiber diet to support digestive health and prevent future flare-ups.

- **High-Fiber Foods**: Fresh fruits and vegetables, whole grains (such as quinoa, farro, and barley), legumes, nuts, and seeds.

- **Varied Protein Sources**: Include lean meats, fish, tofu, and legumes to ensure a balanced intake of nutrients.

General Tips for All Phases

- **Hydration**: Regardless of the phase, staying well-hydrated is crucial. Aim for at least 8 glasses of water a day, more if you're active.

- **Listen to Your Body**: Individual tolerances vary. Use this guide as a starting point and adjust based on your body's responses.

This quick reference guide is intended to be a helpful resource as you manage your diverticulitis through dietary choices. Remember, the key to successful dietary management is flexibility and attentiveness to how foods affect you personally. Always consult with your healthcare provider before making significant changes to your diet, especially during a flare-up.

SCAN HERE TO DOWNLOAD THE BONUSES

OR COPY AND PASTE THE URL:

https://bit.ly/4d3v6Ax